Double Jeopardy

Chronic Mental Illness

Series Editor
John A. Talbott, University of Maryland School of Medicine,
Baltimore, USA

Advisory Board
Leona Bachrach • James T. Barter • Carol Caton • David L. Cutler •
Jeffrey L. Geller • William M. Glazer • Stephen M. Goldfinger •
Howard H. Goldman • H. Richard Lamb • Harriet P. Lefley •
Anthony F. Lehman • Robert P. Lieberman • W. Walter Menninger •
Arthur T. Meyerson

This book is part of a series. The publisher will accept continuation orders which may be cancelled at any time and which provide for automatic billing and shipping of each title in the series upon publication. Please write for details.

Double Jeopardy

Chronic Mental Illness and Substance Use Disorders

Edited by

Anthony F. Lehman

and

Lisa B. Dixon

University of Maryland School of Medicine
Baltimore

 harwood academic publishers

Australia Austria Belgium China France
Germany India Japan Luxembourg Malaysia
Netherlands Russia Singapore Switzerland
Thailand United Kingdom United States

Harwood Academic Publishers
Poststrasse 22
7000 Chur, Switzerland

British Library Cataloguing in Publication Data

Double Jeopardy:Chronic Mental Illness
and Substance Use Disorders. - (Chronic
Mental Illness Series, ISSN 1066-7407;
Vol. 3)
   I. Lehman, Anthony F. II. Dixon, Lisa B.
   III. Series
   616.89

ISBN 3-7186-0599-6

CONTENTS

Section III Social System Issues

INTRODUCTION TO THE SERIES

This series on chronic mental illness is a result of both the success and failure of our efforts over the past thirty years to provide better treatment, rehabilitation and care for persons suffering from severe and persistent mental illnesses. The failure is obvious to all who walk our cities' streets, use our libraries or pass through our transportation terminals. The success is found in the enormous boost of interest in service to, research on and teaching about treatment, rehabilitation and care of those persons who, in Leona Bachrach's definition, "are, have been, or might have been, but for the deinstitutionalization movement, on the rolls of long-term mental institutions, especially state hospitals."

The first book in our modern era devoted to the subject was that by Richard Lamb in 1976, *Community Survival for Long-Term Patients*. Shortly thereafter, Leona Bachrach's unique study "Deinstitutionalization: An Analytical Review and Sociological Perspective" was published. In 1978, the American Psychiatric Association hosted a meeting on the problem that resulted in the publication *The Chronic Mental Patient*. This effort in turn spawned several texts dealing with increasingly specialized areas: *The Chronic Mentally Ill: Treatment, Programs, Systems* and *Chronic Mental Illness in Children and Adolescents*, both by John Looney; and *The Chronic Mental Patient/II* by Walter Menninger and Gerald Hannah.

Now, however, there are a host of publications devoted to various portions of the problem, e.g., the homeless mentally ill, rehabilitation of the mentally ill, families of the mentally ill, and so on. The amount of research and experience now that can be conveyed to a wide population of caregivers is exponentially greater than it was in 1955, the year that deinstitutionalization began.

This series will cover:

— types of intervention, e.g., psychopharmacology, psychotherapy, case management, social and vocational rehabilitation, and mobile and home treatment;

— settings, e.g., hospitals, ambulatory settings, nursing homes, correctional facilities and shelters;

— specific populations, e.g., alcohol and drug abusers, the homeless and those dually diagnosed;

— special issues, e.g., family intervention, psychoeducation, policy/financing, non-compliance, forensic, cross-cultural and systems issues.

I am indebted to our hard-working editorial board as well as to our editors and authors, many of whom are involved in both activities.

This third volume is typical of what we will publish; it covers a specific portion of the field, although overlapping with other books in the series; and it deals with experience, research, intervention strategies and broader social issues. Its editors are both leaders in the area of substance abuse treatment and have the unique ability to bridge the academic and practical worlds.

Future books in this series will cover inpatient care, psychiatric rehabilitation, psychopharmacology, the homeless mentally ill, problems with compliance, alcoholism and drug abuse as chronic conditions and the mentally ill in the correctional system. I hope you will look forward to them as eagerly as I do.

John A. Talbott, MD

CONTRIBUTORS

Theimann Ackerson, MSW, Project Director, New Hampshire–Dartmouth Psychiatric Research Center, Concord, New Hampshire.

Stephen Bartels, MD, Assistant Professor of Clinical Psychiatry, Dartmouth Medical School, Concord, New Hampshire; and Medical Director, West Central Services, Lebanon, New Hampshire.

Melanie Bennett, MS, Doctoral Candidate, Department of Psychology, Rutgers University, New Brunswick, New Jersey.

Kate Bergman Carey, PhD, Associate Professor of Psychology, Department of Psychology, Syracuse University, Syracuse, New York.

Laura M. Champlain, JD, Attorney, Office of the General Counsel, National Security Agency, Fort Mead, Maryland.

Lisa B. Dixon, MD, Assistant Professor of Psychiatry and Medical Director, Assertive Community Treatment Team for Homeless Mentally Ill Persons, Department of Psychiatry, University of Maryland School of Medicine, Baltimore, Maryland.

Robert E. Drake, MD, PhD, Professor of Psychiatry and Director, New Hampshire–Dartmouth, Psychiatric Research Center, Concord, New Hampshire; and Professor of Psychiatry, West Central Services, Lebanon, New Hampshire.

Thomas S. Fox, MD, Medical Director, New Hampshire Division of Mental Health and Developmental Services, Concord, New Hampshire.

Agnes B. Hatfield, PhD, Professor Emeritus, University of Maryland, Baltimore; and founding member of the National Alliance for the Mentally Ill, Greenbelt, Maryland.

Stanley S. Herr, JD, DPhil, Associate Professor of Law, University of Maryland School of Law, Baltimore, Maryland; Kennedy Public Policy Fellow, White House Domestic Policy Council.

Jeannette L. Johnson, PhD, Associate Professor of Psychiatry, University of Maryland School of Medicine, Baltimore, Maryland.

Matthew G. Kushner, PhD, Assistant Professor, Department of Psychiatry, University of Minnesota, Minneapolis, Minnesota.

Anthony F. Lehman, MD, MSPH, Associate Professor of Psychiatry and Director, Center for Mental Health Services Research, Department of Psychiatry, University of Maryland School of Medicine, Baltimore, Maryland.

Joseph Liberto, MD, Chief, Substance Abuse Treatment Program, Baltimore Veterans Administration Medical Center; and Assistant Professor of Psychiatry, University of Maryland at Baltimore, Baltimore, Maryland.

John C. Mahler, MD, Chairman of the Institute of Behavioral Health at Morristown Memorial Hospital, Morristown, New Jersey; and Adjunct Assistant Professor of Psychiatry at Cornell University Medical College, New York, New York. He was formerly Director of the Alcohol Disorders Program at The New York Hospital–Cornell Medical Center, Westchester Division in White Plains, New York.

David McDuff, MD, Associate Professor and Director, Adult and Addiction Psychiatry, Department of Psychiatry, University of Maryland School of Medicine, Baltimore, Maryland.

Carolyn Mercer-McFadden, PhD, Research Associate, New Hampshire–Dartmouth Psychiatric Research Center, Concord, New Hampshire.

Kim T. Mueser, PhD, Associate Professor, Department of Psychiatry, New Hampshire–Dartmouth Psychiatric Research Center, Concord, New Hampshire.

Douglas L. Noordsy, MD, Associate Professor, Department of Psychiatry, Dartmouth Medical School, Clairmont, New Hampshire.

Fred Osher, MD, Director of Community Psychiatry, University of Maryland School of Medicine, Baltimore, Maryland.

Nicole E. Posner, BS, Data Analyst, Department of Psychiatry, University of Maryland School of Medicine, Baltimore, Maryland.

Jill RachBeisel, MD, Assistant Professor of Psychiatry, University of Maryland School of Medicine, Baltimore, Maryland.

M. Susan Ridgely, MSW, JD, Research Associate, Mental Health Policy Studies, Department of Psychiatry, University of Maryland School of Medicine, Baltimore, Maryland.

Jon E. Rolf, PhD, Associate Professor, Department of Maternal and Child Health, School of Public Health and Hygiene, Johns Hopkins University, Baltimore, Maryland.

Robert Schwartz, MD, Assistant Professor of Psychiatry; and Director, University of Maryland Treatment Center, Department of Psychiatry, University of Maryland School of Medicine, Baltimore, Maryland.

Kathleen Sciacca, MA, Executive Director, Sciacca Comprehensive Service Development for Mental Illness, Drug Addiction and Alcoholism (MIDAA), New York, New York.

Donald L. Shumway, MSS, Director, New Hampshire Division of Mental Health and Developmental Services, Concord, New Hampshire.

Roger D. Weiss, MD, Associate Professor of Psychiatry, Harvard Medical School, Belmont, Massachusetts; and Clinical Director of Alcohol and Drug Abuse Program, McLean Hospital, Belmont, Massachusetts.

Joseph Westermeyer, MD, MPH, PhD, Professor of Psychiatry, University of Minnesota, Minneapolis; and Chief, Psychiatry Service, Veterans Affairs Medical Center, Minneapolis, Minnesota.

Eileen J. Wong, MD, Instructor in Psychiatry, Massachusetts Medical Health Center, Boston, Massachusetts.

1

Introduction

ANTHONY F. LEHMAN and LISA B. DIXON

The voices taunt Paul incessantly as they have for years, forcing him to recall horrible past misdeeds, whether real or imagined, he cannot tell. Waves of guilt and depression wrack him. What has he done to deserve this? Attempts over the past few days to drown the tormenting demons with alcohol have provided some hours of relief, only to invite the voices back with even more vengeance. The alcohol no longer provides the escape that it has on so many similar occasions in the past, but the desire to drink is as persistent as the voices. He has tried other escapes — marijuana, downers, even cocaine — but these only make things worse, feeding the voices and driving his family away from him. Paul's desperation now leads him to one painful conclusion — he must kill himself to be free of his living hell. Paul now waits in the emergency room for your evaluation, pacing and talking loudly to himself.

If you are like most mental health or substance abuse clinicians, your first thought may be to try to figure out whether you can refer Paul to someone who is better equipped than you to handle his problems. You then feel helpless that there seems to be no one out there who can help Paul overcome his vicious cycle of mental anguish and substance abuse. He has been to several hospitals, clinics,

1

and drug rehabilitation centers, some of which have helped for a while, but none for very long. Those who have treated Paul have diagnosed him variably as having schizophrenia, organic hallucinosis, alcohol dependence, cocaine dependence, psychotic depression, borderline personality, and antisocial personality. They have given him antipsychotics, antidepressants, lithium, and Antabuse. He has tried treatment free of all substances in a drug rehabilitation program. It seems nearly impossible to know what illnesses Paul has, why he has them, and what he needs to cope with them.

More and more, mental health and substance abuse clinicians are encountering people like Paul in their offices, clinics, hospitals, and treatment centers. It can seem that Paul's problems are too complex for us to help or that the services that Paul needs do not exist. However, out of necessity in recent years, clinicians, researchers, and program planners have been struggling to determine how to help patients like Paul, and these efforts now provide a basis for hope. This book offers a practical examination of the problem of substance disorders among persons with chronic mental illnesses. Our intent is to convey much of what is known in order to assist you with Paul in your office today and to identify what we still must learn so that we can do a better job with the Pauls of tomorrow.

The first section focuses on background and diagnostic issues. How common is the co-occurrence of chronic mental illness and substance use? Are particular mental disorders associated with use of specific drugs? Mueser, Bennett, and Kushner address these questions in Chapter 2 and outline a basic conceptual framework within which we can begin to understand the use of drugs and alcohol by persons with severe mental illnesses. In Chapter 3, Westermeyer then explains significant cultural issues related to the use of substances. The country, the neighborhood, and even the street where an individual lives clearly play a role in every person's decision to use substances. This is no less true for persons with severe and chronic mental illnesses. This chapter equips clinicians with knowledge to understand how these cultural and social factors may influence patients. The last chapter in this section by Drake and Mercer-Mc-Fadden describes the detection and diagnosis of substance disorders in the presence of chronic mental illness. The overlapping symptoms of substance use and mental illness, the cognitive deficits associated with mental illness which impede communication, and denial, each hinders recognition of the problem. This chapter reviews the menu of available strategies and provides clinicians with specific recommendations tailored to their treatment setting.

Building upon this review of the scope of the problem, the cultural context, and the obstacles to its detection, the second section of the book provides practical strategies for treating specific patient subgroups. The heterogeneity of chronic mental illnesses and substance disorders and the range of clinical approaches required throughout the life span renders ineffective any single, uniform approach to *all* patients. However, designing and implementing any treatment for these persons requires a basic vocabulary and repertoire of interventions that draw from both the substance abuse and mental illness fields. All too often, clinicians are comfortable and experienced with one problem, but not the other. The chapter by Schwartz and Lehman first reviews the principles and established techniques for treating chronic mental disorders and substance use disorders when they occur as a single problem. They then summarize the similarities and differences in the treatment of these disorders that must be taken into account when integrating services for dually diagnosed patients. This chapter serves as a reference for subsequent chapters on the treatment of specific patient subgroups.

In their respective chapters, Carey and then Weiss and Wong describe the treatment of substance-using individuals with schizophrenia and mood disorders. Individuals with these disorders have different prognoses, deficits, and patterns of illness and thus require different approaches. The next two chapters, Chapters 8 and 9, focus on both ends of the life span. Substance use and chronic mental disorders often begin during adolescence. Johnson, Posner, and Rolf examine the special needs of these troubled youths and discuss efforts at prevention and early detection. Treatment of the dually diagnosed elderly on the other hand may need to incorporate management of the "end-stage" effects of prolonged comorbidity. Bartels and Liberto explore treatment for this group whose size may increase as the baby boom generation ages and the numbers of elderly persons with chronic mental disorders and substance use grow.

Mahler focuses on another special population, the HIV-infected person with chronic mental illness and substance abuse. Medically vulnerable, this group represents a special challenge both for treatment and prevention. Persons with chronic mental disorders *induced* by substances are the subject of the chapter by RachBeisel and

McDuff. These patients often seek help from the treatment system and suffer from persistent organic mental problems brought on by years of substance use. Are psychopharmacologic and psychosocial interventions the same for these patients as for patients with a primary mental disorder?

Clinical treatment is not delivered in a vacuum. While clinicians have felt confused about how to help persons with chronic mental illness and substance use, social and community systems have also been unprepared. Developing effective treatments for these patients requires involvement of the patient's family and community. The final section of the book explores important aspects of the system context in which treatment must occur. Most persons with chronic mental illness live with their families. Historically blamed for the mental illness of their family members, families have now asserted themselves as knowledgeable and important participants in providing care for their mentally ill loved ones. The additional problem of substance use may make family life even more difficult and frightening. In their chapter, Sciacca and Hatfield present techniques for assessment and intervention with families of dually diagnosed patients.

Because many of these patients can no longer live safely at home, housing looms as a critical issue. Most housing programs for mentally ill persons exclude substance users. Most residential programs for substance abusers do not tolerate those with chronic mental illness. Homelessness often results. Dixon and Osher discuss the problems and potential solutions for housing these persons.

Frequently, dually diagnosed patients end up spending the night in jail rather than at home, in a safe residence or treatment setting. Dually diagnosed individuals are especially vulnerable to running afoul of the legal system, and disturbing evidence mounts that the jails and prisons are substituting for the hospital and other therapeutic alternatives. Furthermore, these patients are in "double jeopardy" because of their dual stigmas, decreasing their access to basic necessities and services. Champlain and Herr discuss the patterns of contacts between dually diagnosed patients and the legal system, the productive and problematic aspects of the relationships between treatment and legal systems, and special considerations regarding advocacy, confidentiality, involuntary treatment, social control, and the promotion of the welfare of both patient and society.

Their notion of "double jeopardy" is so compelling, that we have incorporated it into the title of this book.

The final three chapters address challenges to our current systems of clinical care. Historically, many barriers to providing an adequate level of care to dually diagnosed persons have emerged. Drake, Noordsy and Ackerman explain more optimal coordination of services. The service system, traditionally divided between substance abuse treatment and mental health treatment, requires bridging strategies. Case management and assertive community treatment approaches are emphasized. As system leaders modify the organization of service systems, well-trained personnel must be available to staff these modified systems. Fox and Shumway lay out in Chapter 16 the challenges of training and motivating staff to work with dually diagnosed patients. Finally, Ridgely and Dixon discuss the challenges in public policies that affect the financing and regulation of health care, housing and other human resources and how these must change in order to provide better services for chronically mentally ill persons with substance use disorders.

Although Paul and others like him challenge the limits of our clinical skills and service systems, we hope that this book conveys new knowledge that assists you in caring for such patients. Most important, we would like to convey hope and confidence that treating persons with severe mental illness and substance abuse is worth your time, effort, and perseverance and can make a difference in patients' lives.

Section I:

Background and
Diagnostic Issues

2

Epidemiology of Substance Use Disorders Among Persons with Chronic Mental Illnesses

KIM T. MUESER, MELANIE BENNETT, and MATTHEW G. KUSHNER

In recent years there has been a growing awareness that persons with severe mental illness have an increased risk for the development of substance abuse or dependence disorders compared to the general population. The high vulnerability to alcohol and drug abuse among psychiatric patients presents a myriad of problems to clinicians treating such patients. Patients often deny substance abuse, which may resemble the symptoms of psychiatric disorders, creating diagnostic dilemmas. Furthermore, substance abuse often compromises the protective effects of psychotropic medications, leading to frequent relapses and rehospitalizations. Last, the problem of substance abuse can be frustrating to professionals, who must face the limitations of current treatment options for psychiatric patients with comorbid substance abuse disorders.

In this chapter, we take the first step towards helping clinicians deal more effectively with this pressing problem by reviewing information on the epidemiology of substance abuse in patients with severe mental illness. An understanding of the prevalence of substance abuse in this population and its correlates is necessary in order to facilitate the recognition of patients with these comorbid conditions. We begin with a brief discussion of methodological issues in epidemiological research on substance abuse in psychiatric patients. Next, data on the prevalence of comorbid substance abuse disorders in psychiatric patients is reviewed, as well as the diagnostic and demographic correlates of abuse in this population. Finally, we consider different theories that may account for the high rate of substance abuse in persons with severe mental illness.

METHODOLOGICAL ISSUES

There are several methodological issues which may influence the results of epidemiological studies on the prevalence of substance abuse in psychiatric patients and contribute to the diverse findings in this area, including diagnostic factors, sampling methods, and demographic characteristics.

Diagnostic Factors

Assessing the prevalence of substance abuse in psychiatric patients requires reliable and valid diagnostic methods for each disorder. Studies that employ different definitions of substance abuse naturally will produce prevalence estimates that are difficult to compare. For example, some studies have examined substance *use*, others have focussed on *abuse* or *dependence*, while still others have not specified the definition of substance abuse employed.

A related diagnostic issue is that the methods used to determine diagnoses can influence findings of comorbidity. Diagnoses can be established by structured clinical interviews, non-structured interviews, self-report ratings, and reviews of medical records. Structured clinical interviews generally yield the most reliable diagnoses (Drake, Osher, Noordsy, Hurlbut, Teague & Beaudett, 1990), but not all epidemiological studies of substance abuse in psychiatric patients use such interviews.

In addition, establishing psychiatric diagnoses in patients with comorbid substance abuse may be problematic because the symptoms of substance use and withdrawal can mimic psychiatric disorders (Schuckit, 1983; Schuckit & Monteiro, 1988). For example, chronic alcohol abuse and withdrawal from alcohol can produce psychotic symptoms resembling schizophrenia, as can amphetamine abuse. Alcohol abuse and withdrawal are also associated with increases in depression and anxiety (Kushner, Sher & Beitman, 1990), whereas stimulant abuse and withdrawal from sedatives can lead to panic symptoms and obsessive-compulsive behavior (Schuckit, 1983). Because the symptoms of substance use and withdrawal can resemble psychiatric symptoms, a psychiatric diagnosis can only be confidently established when the patient is not currently abusing alcohol or drugs.

Sampling Methods

The location from which patients are sampled can have an important bearing on estimates of the prevalence of substance abuse in persons with chronic mental illness. For example, surveys conducted in hospital emergency rooms tend to yield higher rates of substance abuse disorders than other settings (Barbee, Clark, Crapanzano, Heintz & Kehoe, 1989; Galanter, Castaneda & Ferman, 1988). Similarly, surveys conducted with psychiatric inpatients may result in lower rates of comorbid substance abuse than outpatients, because severely impaired patients may have less access to drugs or alcohol (Arndt, Tyrell, Flaum & Andreasen, 1992; Cohen & Klein, 1970; Mueser et al., 1990; Mueser, Bellack & Blanchard, 1992-a).

An additional consideration is the population from which the sample is obtained. Estimated rates of comorbidity for any two medical conditions are higher if the sample is drawn from a clinical population (e.g., patients in a hospital or day treatment program) than from the general population (e.g., the community), because of a phenomenon known as "Berkson's fallacy" (Berkson, 1949). This discrepancy is due to the fact that either of the two comorbid disorders may propel patients into treatment, artificially inflating the rate of comorbidity observed in clinical settings. Thus, estimates of the prevalence of substance abuse in severely mentally ill patients based on assessments conducted at treatment settings for these patients tend to be greater than the true prevalence in this population.

Table 2.1. Demographic and Clinical Predictors of
Substance Abuse in Severe Mental Illness

Variable	Correlate with substance abuse
Gender	Male
Age	Young
Education	Low
Premorbid social-sexual adjustment	Good
Age of first hospitalization	Early
Treatment compliance	Poor
Relapse rate	High
Symptom severity	Higher suicidality

Demographic Characteristics

Demographic variables are correlated with substance abuse disorders in the general population and among psychiatric patients. The failure to account for these demographic differences may explain some of the variation in estimates of the prevalence of substance abuse across studies of patients with severe psychiatric disorders (Mueser, Yarnold & Bellack, 1992-b). Key demographic variables that are associated with an increased rate of substance abuse in patients with chronic mental illness are summarized in Table 2.1. For example, young male psychiatric patients are especially prone to develop substance abuse disorders.

PREVALENCE OF SUBSTANCE ABUSE IN PERSONS WITH CHRONIC MENTAL ILLNESS

The ideal sampling method for studying the comorbidity of substance abuse in psychiatric disorders is to assess persons in the community. Using a community sample allows the researcher to avoid the pitfalls of Berkson's fallacy, while controlling for important demographic characteristics such as age and gender. The Epidemiologic Catchment

Area (ECA) study (Regier et al., 1990) represents the largest epidemiological study of psychiatric illness conducted to date, with over 20,000 persons surveyed using structured clinical diagnostic interviews. Although this study combined samples of individuals assessed in the community with samples of psychiatric patients living in hospitals and other treatment settings, it provides the best estimates currently available of the prevalence of comorbid substance abuse in severe psychiatric disorders.

The ECA study provides strong evidence that substance abuse disorders are more prevalent among persons with a mental illness than in the general population. Results of the ECA survey showed that in the general population (i.e., all persons surveyed) the lifetime prevalence for a psychiatric disorder was 22.5%, while the lifetime prevalence for alcohol abuse disorders and drug abuse disorders were 13.5% and 6.1%, respectively. However, among individuals with a psychiatric disorder, 22.3% also had an alcohol abuse disorder, and 14.7% also had a drug abuse disorder. These rates are significantly higher than the base rates found in the general population. In fact, if one compares the lifetime prevalence of substance abuse in persons with no psychiatric illness to that of persons with a psychiatric illness, having a psychiatric disorder more than doubles the chances of a comorbid alcohol abuse diagnosis (11% vs. 22.3%), and increases the chances of a comorbid drug abuse disorder by more than four times (3.7% vs. 14.7%).

Considering the evidence from the ECA study that psychiatric patients are more prone to alcohol and drug abuse, the question arises as to whether some disorders have a higher rate of comorbidity than other disorders. Of special interest is the issue of whether patients with severe mental illness are particularly vulnerable to substance abuse disorders compared to their counterparts with less debilitating illnesses. Once again, the ECA study provides the most data pertaining to these questions.

In addressing this question, we have chosen to focus on DSM-III Axis I disorders, namely schizophrenic, affective, and anxiety disorders. Although some severely mentally ill persons undoubtedly have personality disorders (which are recorded on Axis II of DSM-III), the definitions of some of these disorders clearly overlap with the criteria for substance abuse disorder (e.g., antisocial personality disorder), obscuring a valid estimate of true comorbidity between the disorders. Table 2.2 provides a summary of the prevalence rates of alcohol abuse, drug abuse, and substance abuse disorders (either alcohol and/or drug abuse) for patients with major psychiatric illnesses in the ECA study. This table contains information for each diagnostic group both on the *rate* of substance abuse (i.e., the percentage of patients meeting diagnostic criteria for a substance abuse disorder), as well as the *odds ratio*. The odds ratio is a measure of how much the psychiatric illness increases the chances of also having a substance abuse disorder (e.g., an odds ratio of "2.0" would mean that the mental illness doubles the chances of a comorbid substance abuse disorder, whereas a ratio of "3.0" would reflect a three-fold increased chance).

Inspection of Table 2.2 reveals several interesting trends. First, note that the two psychiatric disorders that are most strongly associated with severe mental illnesses, schizophrenia and bipolar disorder, have the highest rates of comorbid substance abuse. For example, the rate of lifetime substance abuse disorder in schizophrenia was 47.0%, and for bipolar disorder it was 56.1%. This compares to the relatively lower (although still high) rate of substance abuse in major depression (27.2%) or the anxiety disorders (range: 22.9–35.8%). Thus, in addition to the increased risk to substance abuse shared by all psychiatric patients, persons with severe mental illness are especially vulnerable to developing these comorbid disorders.

A second noteworthy trend in Table 2.2 is that the odds ratios for developing a drug abuse disorder, given a psychiatric illness, are consistently greater than the odds ratios for developing a comorbid alcohol abuse disorder. Part of this difference is due to the fact that alcohol abuse disorders are more common than drug abuse disorders. This means that a greater percentage of change is necessary to double the risk (i.e., produce an odds ratio of "2") of developing an alcohol abuse disorder than a drug abuse disorder. However, what this trend also reflects is that having a psychiatric illness, which may be thought of as a type of social deviance, increases the chances of other types of deviant behavior, particularly drug abuse.

The findings of the ECA study that included a large preponderance of persons in the community, are consistent with other reports from treatment settings on the prevalence of substance abuse in persons with severe mental illness. For example, Mueser et al. (1990) reported that in a sample of 149 schizophrenia-spectrum disorder patients receiving inpatient treatment for an acute symptom

Table 2.2. Lifetime Prevalence (%) and Odds
Ratios (OR) of Substance Use Disorder
for Various Psychiatric Disorders

Psychiatric disorder	Any substance abuse or dependence		Any alcohol diagnosis		Any drug diagnosis	
	%	OR	%	OR	%	OR
General population	16.7	–	13.5	–	6.1	–
Schizophrenia	47.0	4.6	33.7	3.3	27.5	6.2
Any affective disorder	32.0	2.6	21.8	1.9	19.4	4.7
Any bipolar disorder	56.1	6.6	43.6	5.1	33.6	8.3
Major depression	27.2	1.9	16.5	1.3	18.0	3.8
Dysthymia	31.4	2.4	20.9	1.7	18.9	3.9
Any anxiety disorder	23.7	1.7	17.9	1.5	11.9	2.5
Obsessive-compulsive disorder	32.8	2.5	24.0	2.1	18.4	3.7
Phobia	22.9	1.6	17.3	1.4	11.2	2.2
Panic disorder	35.8	2.9	28.7	2.6	16.7	3.2

Odds ratios = ratio of the odds of having the substance use disorder in the psychiatric diagnostic group to the odds of the disorder in the remaining population. Based on data from the
National Institute of Mental Health Epidemiological Catchment
Area Study (Regier et al., 1990).

exacerbation, 47% had a life-time diagnosis of alcohol abuse, while
many also had abused cannabis (42%), stimulants (25%), and hallucinogens (18%). Barbee et al. (1989) found comparable rates of
substance abuse among schizophrenic patients presenting at a crisis
service: 47% met criteria for a lifetime diagnosis of alcohol abuse,
while 37% had histories of drug abuse. Similar rates for patients with
schizophrenia have been reported in other studies as well (e.g., O'-

Farrell, Connors & Upper, 1983; Dixon, Haas, Weiden, Sweeney & Frances, 1991). Furthermore, the rates found in the ECA study are also in line with other studies of the prevalence of substance abuse in bipolar disorder (reviewed by Goodwin and Jamison, 1990), major depression (e.g., Merikangas, Leckman, Prusoff & Weissman, 1985; Lewis, Rice, Andreasen, Endicott & Hartman, 1986), and anxiety disorders (reviewed by Kushner, 1990).

As might be expected, surveys of substance abuse in persons with severe mental illness suggest similar or even higher rates to those reported for patients with schizophrenia and bipolar disorders in the ECA study. For example, Ananth, Vandewater, Kamal, Brodsky, Garnal and Miller (1989) reported that 72% of a sample of persons with schizophrenia, bipolar disorder, or atypical psychosis had a history of substance abuse. Similarly, McClellan, Druley and Carson (1978) and Safer et al. (1987) reported that 49% and 73%, respectively, of their samples of severe psychiatric patients had histories of substance abuse. In sum, clinicians who treat persons with severe mental illness should expect that about half of their patients will have a positive history of substance abuse. In addition, most surveys suggest that about half of the patients with a history of substance abuse (i.e., 25% of all severly mentally ill persons) have a *current* drug or alcohol abuse problem (e.g., Mueser et al., 1990; Noordsy et al., 1991).

SPECIFIC PATTERNS OF SUBSTANCE ABUSE IN PSYCHIATRIC PATIENTS

The issue of whether psychiatric patients demonstrate a preference for specific classes of substances has been debated for more than a decade. As will be discussed in more detail in the next section, self-medication of psychiatric symptoms has been advanced as an explanation for the high rate of substance abuse in persons with severe mental illness (e.g., Khantzian, 1985). According to this hypothesis, some patients select specific drugs to counteract the dysphoric experience associated with particular symptoms. For example, persons with schizophrenia have been reported to be especially prone to abuse stimulants (reviewed by Schneier and Siris, 1987), presumably to counteract the effects of negative symptoms, whereas patients with bipolar disorders may selectively use alcohol to treat manic states (Hensel, Dunner & Fieve, 1979).

Despite the intuitive appeal of theories that suggest the drug choice of psychiatric patients is based on the specific effects of the substance, the data supporting preferential drug selection is slim at best. In a relatively large survey of 263 briefly hospitalized psychiatric inpatients with diagnoses of schizophrenia, schizoaffective disorder, bipolar disorder, and major depression, Mueser et al. (1992-b) found little difference between the groups in the specific substances of choice. Furthermore, over an eight year period, significant changes were found in the drug abuse patterns of the patients with schizophrenic and schizoaffective disorders, with cannabis abuse declining and cocaine increasing in a fashion comparable to the general population (Mueser et al., 1992-b). Similarly, the ECA study also failed to find significant differences between diagnostic groups in terms of vulnerability to specific drug types. The available data suggest that at this time, demographic variables are more important determinants than clinical variables (e.g., diagnosis) of which specific substances are abused by psychiatric patients. Thus, in two studies conducted at the Medical College of Pennsylvania, we found that age (youth) was a strong predictor of stimulant abuse, whereas low socioeconomic status (SES) predicted abuse of illicit drugs (cannabis, cocaine) and high SES predicted abuse of prescription tranquilizers (Mueser et al., 1990; 1992-b).

Rather than epidemiological research pointing to specific drug preferences in mentally ill persons, the evidence suggests that the substance abuse behavior of these patients frequently spans across a range of different drug classes, with polydrug abuse often the norm in urban settings where alcohol as well as a variety of illicit drugs are available. Chen and collegues (1992) found that one-third of their sample of psychiatric inpatients in an inner city hospital were polydrug abusers, a finding mirrored by other studies that have reported a predilection for psychiatric patients in or near cities to abuse a variety of different drugs (e.g., Cohen & Klein, 1970; Mueser et al., 1990). In contrast, Noordsy et al. (1991) reported that only 13.3% of patients with schizophrenia living in a rural setting had a history of drug abuse, compared to 50.7% with a history of alcohol abuse. Taken together, these findings indicate that persons with severe mental illness are prone to abusing those substances which are most available to them. In almost all studies alcohol is the substance most commonly abused, followed by whatever illicit drug is most popular at the time.

MODELS LINKING MENTAL ILLNESS AND SUBSTANCE ABUSE

The high prevalence of substance abuse in psychiatric patients raises the fundamental question of what accounts for this increased rate of comorbidity? Kushner and Mueser (in press), among others (Meyer, 1986; Lehman, Myers & Corty, 1989; Anthony, 1991), have suggested that there are four possible general models that can account for the increased rate of comorbid substance abuse in psychiatric patients: 1) the secondary substance abuse model; 2) the secondary psychiatric disorder model; 3) the common factor model; and 4) the bidirectional model. Each of these models is described below, followed by a brief consideration of the data supporting it.

The Secondary Substance Abuse Model

According to this model, higher than expected rates of comorbidity are the result of the mental illness increasing patients' vulnerability to substance abuse. Consistent with this model, some research suggests that the onset of chronic and severe psychiatric illnesses predates the onset of substance abuse disorders. For example, Powell, Read, Penicky, Miller and Bingham (1987) found that in a large sample of veterans with alcoholism and psychiatric disorders, 59% reported that psychiatric problems began first, 22% said the onset of the psychiatric and substance abuse problems coincided, and 19% reported the alcohol problems began first. However, the data from other studies are mixed with respect to how often anxiety disorders and depression precede the development of substance abuse disorders (Hesselbrock, Meyers & Keener, 1985; Christie, Burke, Regier, Rae, Boyd & Locke, 1988; Ross, Glaser & Germason, 1988).

The notion that psychiatric illness leads to substance abuse in many patients has intuitive appeal to clinicians, because patients are usually able to give coherent reasons for their substance abuse. Most of the reasons patients with severe mental illness give for using alcohol or drugs (Test, Wallisch, Allness & Ripp, 1989; Dixon, Haas, Weiden, Sweeney & Frances, 1990, 1991; Noordsy et al., 1991) are similar to the reasons or expectations of primary substance abusers with no comorbid psychiatric disorder (Brown, Millar & Passman,

1988; Cooper, Russell, Skinner & Windle, 1992). These reasons can be divided into three major categories:

Self-medication of negative affective states. Persons with severe mental disorders experience high levels of anxiety, depression, apathy, and frustration, negative moods which may increase their propensity to use alcohol or drugs to escape or mollify these feelings.

Social facilitation. Persons with severe mental illness typically have fewer available social outlets than non-impaired individuals. Since the majority of substance abuse among psychiatric patients occurs in a social setting (Dixon et al., 1990), using drugs or alcohol with others may be a convenient outlet for meeting their social needs. Furthermore, social groups of substance abusers tend to have a higher tolerance for deviant behavior in its members, and belonging to such a group may help psychiatric patients gain acceptance and identity independent of their illness (Lamb, 1982).

Pleasure enhancement. Similar to the "Social Facilitation" explanation, persons with chronic mental illness tend to have fewer opportunities to experience pleasure, and the use of drugs or alcohol may provide an easy and rapid solution to this need.

The empirical support for each of these explanations at this time relies mainly on the face validity of the verbal reports of psychiatric patients. Studies that have compared the symptom severity of patients with versus without a history of substance abuse have failed to find consistent differences (e.g., Bernadt and Murray, 1986; Barbee et al., 1989; Mueser et al., 1990; Dixon et al., 1991). However, these negative findings cannot rule out the validity of the explanations patients give for their substance abuse. Future research is needed in this area to explore whether a link can be established between the specific reasons psychiatric patients give for using drugs and alcohol, and independent measures of their symptomatology and social drive. Such research will provide a test of the hypothesis that these reasons for abuse account for the increased prevalence of substance abuse in persons with chronic mental illness.

The Secondary Psychiatric Disorder Model

This model posits that some cases of psychiatric illness develop as a consequence of substance abuse. Although in many individuals with severe mental illness, the substance abuse precedes the onset of the psychiatric disorder, some research suggests that the substance abuse may have precipitated an existing psychobiological vulnerability, rather than actually *causing* the disorder. Tsuang, Simpson and Kranfol (1982) found few differences between psychotic patients admitted with a recent history of substance abuse and patients with schizophrenia with no history of abuse. Similarly, Vardy and Kay (1983) concluded that LSD was capable of precipitating psychotic reactions only in persons with a vulnerability to psychosis.

On the other hand, there is intriguing epidemiological research from both the ECA study (Tien & Anthony, 1990) and Sweden (Andersson, Allebect, Engstrom & Rydbery, 1987) indicating that alcohol and drug use is predictive of an increased risk of later psychotic symptoms and disorders. These surveys are based on large numbers of persons and do not permit a disentangling of the "chicken and the egg" problem. That is, individuals who are more prone to substance use may have already begun to experience mild levels of psychiatric symptoms that coincide with or precede substance abuse. Nevertheless, this research suggests the possibility that substance abuse may play a role in the etiology of some cases of chronic mental illness.

The Common Factor Model

According to this model, the increased rate of comorbidity between mental illness and substance abuse can be attributed to a common third variable. The candidate for a "third variable" that has been most extensively studied has been genetic vulnerability, which has been examined by patterns of cross-generational transmission of psychiatric and substance abuse disorders in families. Although there is evidence indicating that patients with severe mental and substance abuse disorders are more likely to have relatives with histories of substance abuse (Tsuang et al., 1982; Vardy & Kay, 1983; Gershon et al., 1988), family studies strongly suggest that vulnerability to mental illness is not associated with an increased rate of substance abuse disorders in the relatives of patients (Kendler, 1985; Merikangas & Gelernter, 1990).

It appears that familial factors may contribute independently to a risk for psychiatric or substance abuse disorders, but that such factors do not account for a shared etiologic substrate for both conditions, and therefore cannot explain the increased rate of comorbidity.

It is possible that other, non-genetic common factors exist which increase vulnerability to both mental illness and substance abuse. Socioenvironmental stress (e.g., poverty, unemployment), poor social competence, and neurological "soft signs" are examples of such common factors which may increase the risk of either type of disorder. The role of such common factors in accounting for the high rate of comorbidity between substance abuse and mental illness remains to be examined.

The Bidirectional Model

The bidirectional model stipulates that substance abuse and mental illness interact so that either disorder can initiate or influence the other. Because of the numerous possible permutations of this model, little research currently exists that tests its validity. However, there are many reasons to suspect that substance abuse behavior interacts with severe mental illness to produce a high rate of comorbidity. Consistent with their self-reports, psychiatric patients may use drugs and alcohol to achieve short-term improvements in negative emotions and social contacts, but may pay the long-term cost of a worsening of their mental illness (Drake & Wallach, 1989). Consistent with this, most patients with schizophrenia and alcohol abuse disorders report using alcohol to alleviate anxiety and depression, and to enhance pleasure and social contacts, but not to treat their psychotic symptoms (Noordsy et al., 1991).

Additional factors which may interact with one another include unemployment and impairments in social competence, both of which are associated with substance abuse disorders and mental illness. The bidirectional model appreciates that multiple pathways to comorbidity may be present across different individuals and different diagnoses, and that comorbid conditions, once established, may be interactive and mutually maintaining (Kushner & Mueser, 1993).

CONCLUSIONS

Research on the epidemiology of substance abuse disorders in persons with chronic mental illness indicates a high prevalence of these disorders, with most estimates ranging between 40% and 60%. Demographic characteristics of the patients, rather than clinical features of their illness (e.g., diagnosis, symptom severity), tend to be more predictive of which patients are prone to substance abuse and which specific types of substances will be used. The reason for the high rate of comorbidity between psychiatric illness and substance abuse disorders is not well understood at this time. Models that suggest substance abuse is secondary to psychiatric illness (i.e., patients use substances to self-medicate symptoms, enhance pleasure, and facilitate social interactions), but recognize that substance abuse and mental illness can be mutually maintaining, appear to have the most promise for understanding the relationship between the two conditions. It is likely that multiple pathways exist between substance abuse and severe mental illness, and evaluating which pathways are crucial for which patients will be necessary in optimizing treatments for this difficult population.

REFERENCES

Ananth, J., Vandewater, S., Kamal, M., Brodsky, A., Gamal, R., & Miller, M. (1989). Mixed diagnosis of substance abuse in psychiatric patients. *Hospital and Community Psychiatry. 40,* 297–299.

Andersson, S., Allebeck, P., Engstrom, A., & Rydberg, V. (1987). Cannabis and schizophrenia: A longitudinal study of Swedish conscripts. *Lancet.* December 26, 1483–1486.

Anthony, J.C. (1991). Epidemiology of drug dependence and illicit drug use. *Current Opinion in Psychiatry. 4,* 435–439.

Arndt, S., Tyrrell, G., Flaum, M., & Andreasen, N.C. (1992). Comorbidity of substance abuse and schizophrenia: The role of pre-morbid adjustment. *Psychological Medicine. 22,* 379–388.

Barbee, J.G., Clark, P.D., Crapanzano, M.S., Heintz, G.C., & Kehoe, C.E. (1989). Alcohol and substance abuse among schizophrenic patients presenting to an emergency psychiatric service. *Journal of Nervous and Mental Disease. 177,* 400–407.

Berkson, J. (1949). Limitations of the application of four-fold tables to hospital data. *Biometric Bulletin. 2,* 47–53.

Bernadt, M.W., & Murray, R.M. (1986). Psychiatric disorder, drinking, and alcoholism: What are the links? *British Journal of Psychiatry. 148,* 393–400.

Brown, S.A., Millar, A., & Passman, L. (1988). Utilizing expectancies in alcoholism treatment. *Psychology of Addictive Behavior. 2*, 59–65.

Chen, C., Balogh, R., Bathija, J., Howanitz, E., Plutchik, R., & Conte, H.R. (1992). Substance abuse among psychiatric inpatients. *Comprehensive Psychiatry. 33*, 60–64.

Christie, K.A., Burke, J.D., Regier, D.A., Rae, D.S., Boyd, J.H., & Locke, B.Z. (1988). Epidemiologic evidence for early onset of mental disorders and higher risk of drug abuse in young adults. *American Journal of Psychiatry. 145*, 971–975.

Cohen, M., & Klein, D.F. (1970). Drug abuse in a young psychiatric population. *American Journal of Orthopsychiatry. 40*, 448–455.

Cooper, M.L., Russell, M., Skinner, J.B., & Windle, M. (1992). Development and validation of a three-dimensional measure of drinking motives. *Psychological Assessment. 4*, 123–132.

Dixon, L., Haas, G., Weiden, P., Sweeney, J., & Frances, A. (1990). Acute effects of drug abuse in schizophrenic patients: Clinical observations and patients' self-reports. *Schizophrenia Bulletin. 16*, 69–79.

Dixon, L., Haas, G., Weiden, P., Sweeney, J., & Frances, A. (1991). Drug abuse in schizophrenic patients: Clinical correlates and reasons for use. *American Journal of Psychiatry. 148*, 224–230.

Drake, R.E., & Wallach, M.A. (1989). Substance abuse among the chronically mentally ill. *Hospital and Community Psychiatry. 40*, 1041–1046.

Drake, R.E., Osher, F.C., Noordsy, D.L., Hurlbut, S.C., Teague, G.B., & Beaudett, M.S., (1990). Diagnosis of alcohol use disorders in schizophrenia. *Schizophrenia Bulletin. 16*, 57–67.

Galanter, M., Castaneda, R., & Ferman, J. (1988). Substance abuse among general psychiatric patients: Place of presentation, diagnosis, and treatment. *American Journal of Drug and Alcohol Abuse. 14*, 211–235.

Gershon, E.S., DeLisi, L.E., Hamovit, J., Nurhberger, J.I., Jr., Maxwell, M.E., Schreiber, J., Dauphinais, D., Dingman, C.W., II, & Guroff, J.J. (1988). A controlled family study of chronic psychosis. *Archives of General Psychiatry. 45*, 328–336.

Goodwin, F.K., & Jamison, K.R. (1990). *Manic-Depressive Illness.* New York: Oxford University Press.

Hensel, B., Dunner, D.L., & Fieve, R.R. (1979). The relationship of family history of alcoholism to primary affective disorder. *Journal of Affective Disorders. 1*, 105–113.

Hesselbrock, M.N., Meyer, R.E., & Keener, J.J. (1985). Psychopathology in hospitalized alcoholics. *Archives of General Psychiatry. 42*, 1050–1055.

Kendler, K.S. (1985). A twin study of individuals with both schizophrenia and alcoholism. *British Journal of Psychiatry. 147*, 48–53.

Khantzian, E.J. (1985). The self-medication hypothesis of addictive disorders: Focus on heroin and cocaine dependence. *American Journal of Psychiatry.* 142, 1259–1264.

Kushner, M.G., & Mueser, K.T. (1993). Psychiatric co-morbidity with alcohol disorders (pp. 37–59). In: *Eighth Special Report to the U.S. Congress on Alcohol and Health.* Rockville, MD: U.S. Department of Health and Human Services (NIH Pub. No. 94-3699).

Kushner, M.G., Sher, K.J., & Beitman, B.D. (1990). The relation between alcohol problems and the anxiety disorders. *American Journal of Psychiatry.* 147, 685–695.

Lamb, H.R. (1982). Young adult chronic patients: The new drifters. *Hospital and Community Psychiatry.* 33, 465–468.

Lehman, A.F., Myers, C.P., & Corty E. (1989). Assessment and classification of patients with psychiatric and substance abuse syndromes. *Hospital and Community Psychiatry.* 40, 1019–1025.

Lewis, C.E., Rice, J., Andreasen, N., Endicott, J., & Hartman, A. (1986). Clinical and family correlates of alcoholism in men with unipolar major depression. *Alcoholism: Clinical and Experimental Research.* 10(6), 657–662.

McLellan, A.T., Druley, K.A., & Carson, J.E. (1978). Evaluation of substance abuse problems in a psychiatric hospital. *Journal of Clinical Psychiatry.* 39, 425–430.

Merikangas, K.R., & Gelernter, C.S. (1990). Comorbidity for alcoholism and depression. *Psychiatric Clinics of North America.* 13, 613–632.

Merikangas, K.R., Leckman, J.F., Prusoff, B.A., Pauls, D.L., & Weissman, M.M. (1985). Familial transmission of depression and alcoholism. *Archives of General Psychiatry.* 42, 367–372.

Meyer, R.E. (1986). How to understand the relationship between psychopathology and addictive disorders: Another example of the chicken and the egg. In R.E. Meyer (Ed.), *Psychopathology and Addictive Disorders* (pp. 3–16). New York: Guilford Press.

Mueser, K.T., Bellack, A.S., & Blanchard, J.J. (1992-a). Comorbidity of schizophrenia and substance abuse: Implications for treatment. *Journal of Consulting and Clinical Psychology.* 60, 845–856.

Mueser, K.T., Yarnold, P.R., & Bellack, A.S. (1992-b). Diagnostic and demographic correlates of substance abuse in schizophrenia and major affective disorders. *Acta Psychiatrica Scandinavica.* 85, 48–55.

Mueser, K.T., Yarnold, P.R., Levinson, D.F., Singh, H., Bellack, A.S., Kee, K., Morrison, R.L., & Yadalam, K.G. (1990). Prevalence of substance abuse in schizophrenia: Demographic and clinical correlates. *Schizophrenia Bulletin.* 16, 31–56.

Noordsy, D.L., Drake, R.E., Teague, G.B., Osher, F.C., Hurlbut, S.C., Beaudett, M.S., & Paskus, T.S. (1991). Subjective experiences related to alcohol use among schizophrenics. *Journal of Nervous and Mental Disease. 179*, 410–414.

O'Farrell, T.J., Connors, G.J., & Upper, D. (1983). Addictive behaviors among hospitalized psychiatric patients. *Addictive Behaviors. 8*, 329–333.

Powell, B.J., Read, M.R., Penick, E.C., Miller, N.S., & Bingham, S.F. (1987). Primary and secondary depression in alcoholic men: An important distinction? *Journal of Clinical Psychiatry. 46*, 98–101.

Regier, D.A., Farmer, M.E., Rae, D.S., Locke, B.Z., Keith, S.J., Judd, L.L., & Goodwin, F.K. (1990). Comorbidity of mental disorders with alcohol and other drug abuse: Results from the Epidemiologic Catchment Area (ECA) Study. *Journal of the American Medical Association. 264*, 2511–2518.

Ross, H.E., Glaser, F.B., & Germanson, T. (1988). The prevalence of psychiatric disorders in patients with alcohol and other drug problems. *Archives of General Psychiatry. 45*, 1023–1031.

Safer, D.J. (1987). Substance abuse by young adult chronic patients. *Hospital and Community Psychiatry. 38*, 511–514.

Schneier, F.R., & Siris, S.G. (1987). A review of psychoactive substance use and abuse in schizophrenia: Patterns of drug choice. *Journal of Nervous and Mental Disease. 175*, 641–650.

Schuckit, M.A. (1983). Alcoholism and other psychiatric disorders. *Hospital and Community Psychiatry. 34*, 1022–1027.

Schuckit, M.A., & Monteiro, M.G. (1988). Alcoholism, anxiety, and depression. *British Journal of Addiction. 83*, 1373–1380.

Test, M.A., Wallisch, L.S., Allness, D.J., & Ripp, K. (1989). Substance use in young adults with schizophrenic disorders. *Schizophrenia Bulletin. 15*, 465–476.

Tien, A.Y., & Anthony, J.C. (1990). Epidemiological analysis of alcohol and drug use as risk factors for psychotic experiences. *Journal of Nervous and Mental Disease. 178*, 473–480.

Tsuang, M.T., Simpson, J.C., & Kronfol, Z. (1982). Subtypes of drug abuse with psychosis. *Archives of General Psychiatry. 39*, 141–147.

Vardy, M.M., & Kay, S.R. (1983). LSD psychosis or LSD induced schizophrenia. *Archives of General Psychiatry. 40*, 877–883.

3

Ethnic and Cultural Factors in Dual Disorders

JOSEPH WESTERMEYER

INTRODUCTION

Reports in the scientific literature regarding comorbid psychoactive substance use and psychiatric disorders have been increasing over the last several years. However, the number of such reports that include data or analysis of ethnic and cultural factors is small. Moreover, the definitions of terms, sampling methods, and methods of data collection in such studies varies considerably. Even finding such studies poses a notable task, since relevant articles are sparsely distributed across scores of anthropologic, epidemiologic, medical, psychiatric, and substance abuse journals and books. Thus, *meta-analysis* of the literature is not easily accomplished. Inevitably, one must call upon clinical and research experience, as well as publications, in crafting an overview on this topic, about which much more needs to be learned. This introduces the opportunity for creativity as well as bias in linking culture to comorbid psychopathology.

Differences in *quantitative rates* of medical pathology across ethnicities and cultures are the rule rather than the exception. Causes for such diversity can include genetic factors (e.g., sickle cell disease) as well as environmental factors (e.g., infectious agents, nutrition, finances, public security, education). Indeed, the narrow distribution of schizophrenia, and other psychiatric disorders across ethnicities and cultures is an exception rather than the rule in comparative studies. Unlike rates of schizophrenia across groups, rates of substance use disorders vary widely. Whether the *qualitative* nature of comorbid psychiatric and substance disorders also varies is unknown, although clinicians certainly observe very similar comorbid conditions across greatly different groups.

Culture refers to the total physical, psychosocial, and sociopolitical lifeway of a group of people. It includes the technological resources utilized by them, their dress, housing, means of production and transportation. Cultural lifeways differ in their methods of child raising and education, their means of assigning social role and status, their ways of organizing and governing themselves, and their closely held values and attitudes. Cultural elements, such as skill in technological areas, valued endeavors and status, tend to be integrated internally with each other. In regard to psychoactive substances, choice and pattern of substance use tend to be related to valued psychological states and experiences, economic forces, community values, laws and law enforcement.

Ethnicity refers to diversity of characterisitics among groups living within a distinct geo-political system. These groups typically share mass media, are subject to the same laws and government, and have the same or similar educational system. They may work in the same places, enjoy leisure time in similar ways, shop in the same stores and live in the same or adjacent neighborhoods. Cultural and racial factors may favor different identities despite these similarities, however. Ethnic identity encompasses race, religion, national origin, dress, primary language (even though a *lingua franca* may be spoken in public settings), child raising, family organization, modes of recreation, political affiliations and economic endeavors. Such differences within a multiethnic community or nation-state can produce considerable mischief. For example, a majority of the people may decide that a certain drug is illicit, even though that drug may be acceptable to a minority ethnic group. Impoverished ethnic groups may accept illicit drug production or commerce as an acceptable economic means for survival, although mainstream groups may find this activity to be unacceptable. Mainstream groups may enforce anti-drug laws more stringently in some ethnic neighborhoods than in others.

Everyone belongs to a culture and manifests ethnic values, attitudes, and behaviors, including professionals and researchers in the mental illness-substance disorder field. These cultural and ethnic features of one's *identity* inevitably pull the individual towards some groups, values, and behaviors, and pushes that person away from others. To some extent, advanced education, training and life experiences tend to homogenize individuals. Thus, university trained professionals and researchers, who work in similar fields and have lived in more than one culture, tend to affiliate with one another, at times even more than with members of their own ethnic group. Still, ethnic factors can override these professional affiliations and identities.

Dual disorder may refer to numerous comorbid conditions, such as more than one psychoactive substance use disorder (PSUD) diagnosis, or a PSUD diagnosis plus an Axis 3 bio-medical condition. In this discussion, however, dual disorder refers to comorbid PSUD and Axis I chronic mental illness (CMI). Because so little is known about ethnicity factors related to dual diagnosis, this chapter focuses on ethnic and cultural influences on substance use and abuse with the assumption that these influences apply to persons with mental illnesses as well as the general population.

DIFFERENCES IN ENSOCIALIZING CHILDREN TO SUBSTANCE USE

Cultural and ethnic groups can affect the comorbidity of PSUD and SMI through their *ensocialization* of children, adolescents and young adults. This cultural influence can be accomplished through proscribing the use of certain psychoactive substances, or prescribing their use in particular safe and stereotypic ways. As we shall see, however, these methods do not necessarily operate as deterrents if individuals leave their cultural or ethnic group. Use of psychoactive agents outside of those proscribed and prescribed ways can carry risk of PSUD.

An outstanding example of a group that proscribes virtually all recreational or self-prescribed psychoactive substances are the Mormons. As long as adherents remain active in and faithful to the Mormon faith, abuse of alcohol, tobacco, caffeine (at least in its traditional forms, such as coffee), and other drugs is virtually absent. However, those Mormons who leave the group of faithful practitioners are at risk of PSUD (Eaton & Weil, 1955).

Similarly, many American Indian tribes have anti-alcohol prohibition laws on their reservations and raise their children to value abstinence from alcohol. Nonetheless, many American Indians who choose to drink despite their tribal proscriptions are afflicted with PSUD (Westermeyer, 1974-a). Other American Indians drink moderately on ritual occasions, much as do many other Americans.

A similar effect of parental acculturation on youthful drug use, abuse and abstinence has also been observed among Hispanic American youths (Gfroerer & DeLaRosa, 1993). In a study of Asian, Black, Hispanic and White adolescents in the United States, Maddahian, Newcomb, and Bentler (1986) found other variables to be stronger than ethnicity, including availability of drugs among friends, ease of acquisition of drugs, and earned income to purchase drugs.

Numerous Islamic societies proscribe the use of alcohol, with greater or lesser rigor. In some Islamic societies, the proscription remains a moral-religious one, whereas in theocratic Islamic societies the proscription carries the weight of secular law, which is at times strict, even severe. In general, alcoholism is infrequent in Islamic societies, but can be seen somewhat more often in societies which tolerate use despite religious strictures. Of interest, many Islamic societies abide use and even abuse of other substances. These include not only use of tobacco and caffeine-containing substances, but also use and abuse of cannabis, opiates and other substances. Indeed, the opium-producing Golden Crescent ranges through the Islamic countries of Bangladesh, Pakistan, Afghanistan, Iran and Turkey (Westermeyer, 1983).

Perhaps more common is the prescribing of certain psychoactive substance use in religious ceremonials, family rituals, communal celebrations, as well as "time out" recreation. Typically this involves teaching children or adolescents to use the substance, often in a multigenerational family setting. Adults usually control dosing (such as number of drinks) so that the initiate has a satisfactory experience, and does not come to dislike the psychoactive experience. Other characteristics of this "social prescription" method include the following:

- mandatory use or "the imperative" to use (i.e., opting out is not an option);

- use outside of prescribed times or in excess of prescribed amounts is condemned as inimical to or outside of the cultural/ethnic group.

This strategy tends to be highly effective in reducing or eliminating PSUD.

One method of ensocialization often conducive to subsequent PSUD involves peer introduction to psychoactive substance use. Typically, this begins sometimes between late childhood and early adulthood. Slightly older males introduce slightly younger males and females to use, often in a surreptitious setting (especially if it involves either an illicit substance or under-age use of a legal substance). Use tends to be rapid, with intoxication (rather than sociability or ritual celebration) as the goal. Unlike ceremonial or ritual use, which often involves eating or feasting, peer initiation rarely involves eating.

Most ensocialization occurs within the family, although community, mass media and other social influences play a role. Family influence over substance use may differ among ethnic groups. For example, in a study of father-offspring tobacco smoking congruence, Whites showed a significantly greater congruence than did Blacks (Bauman, Foshee, Linzer, & Koch, 1990).

Ensocialization may occur through formal education of children in such institutions as schools, religious or health facilities. It appears that children in the United States have poor understanding of the psychoactive properties of alcohol, regardless of ethnicity (Giacopassi & Stein, 1991).

CULTURAL AND ETHNIC INFLUENCES ON SUBSTANCE USE

Choice of Substance, Pattern of Use, History of Use

Examples exist of increased rates of CMI in certain ethnic/cultural groups in association with abuse of particular substances. For example, Padilla, Ramirez, Morales, and Olmedo (1977) have found increased rates of mental retardation among children in communities plagued by childhood abuse of *volatile inhalants*. These communities include a section of Mexico City and certain American Indian reservations in Southwestern United States. Recently, inhalant abuse has been reported in areas of Asia, such as Singapore (Teck-Hong, 1986), suggesting that poverty alone does not foster inhalant abuse. Among a group of American Indian students, increased inhalant abuse has been related to lower mathematics scores and written language scores on a standardized test, lower grade point averages, fewer social assets, and lower self-appraisal (Wingert & Fifield, 1985).

Alcohol-related psychopathology has been noted among first and second generation Irish immigrants in two settings. These include New York (Roberts & Myers, 1967) and the United Kingdom during the mid-1900's. A frequent Irish pattern has consisted of tavern-centered drinking throughout an entire evening, sometimes to the point of intoxication. Local taverns substitute for the home and church as a locus of social affiliation, especially among immigrants away from home.

Choice of intoxicant can change over time. For example, traditional kava use among Native Hawaiians has largely given way to "water from America," or alcohol (Keaulana & Whitney, 1990). Kava was known to produce addictive use and certain bio-medical conditions of the eyes and skin, but it was not known to produce or be associated with CMI.

It could be surmised that certain racial groups deficient in *aldehyde dehydrogenase* would be protected against alcohol abuse, and subsequent associated CMI. However, its protective abilities are at best limited, and possibly nonexistent. For example, about twenty-five percent of Koreans are deficient in the enzyme. Nonetheless, their prevalence of alcohol abuse is higher than that of Americans (Lee et al., 1990).

Binge drinking is considerably more likely to produce trauma as well as psychiatric complications and hospitalization (Isreal et al., 1991). These conditions include both acute, often recurrent conditions, such as delirium tremens and alcoholic hallucinosis, as well as chronic, irreversible conditions, such as alcohol amnestic disorder and alcoholic dementia. In a comparison of American Indian and other patients with PSUD, the American Indians were noted to have more of both the acute, recurrent mental disorders as well as more chronic mental disorder (Westermeyer, 1993).

In a survey of alcohol use among Black and White youths who drank heavily, Ringwalt and Palmer (1990) observed that White youth drank more heavily. Ethnic-related *beliefs* and *attitudes* were related to this difference in drinking amounts. Black youth were more apt to believe that drunkenness would lead to health problems and that alcohol was addicting. White youths were less concerned about their parents' opinions regarding their drinking and more concerned about disapproval of their peers.

Some data indicates that *historical factors* may influence a culture's use or abuse of alcohol. For example, aboriginal peoples in America and Australia presumably learned a style of drinking associated with lower class European seamen, traders and adventurers, living in a predominantly male society, with violence, gambling, drunkenness, and sexual license as the norm (Brady, 1990; MacAndrew & Edgerton, 1969). Thus, the men in these societies may have simply emulated the style of intoxication that they observed among a people whose technology, religion, clothes, and other characteristics they were assuming in a period of rapid cultural change.

Carpenter and Ewing (1989) have posited an inverse relationship between the *historical experience* with alcohol (in years or centuries) within a society and the prevalence of alcoholism in the society. Indeed, there are much data to support their notion. Examples include the low rates of alcoholism among the Chinese (at least until opium addiction was stifled), South Asian Hindu and Moslem societies (both of which have religious strictures against alcohol), and para-Mediterranean peoples (where ceremonial and ritual drinking has been known for millennia). Nonetheless, there are examples to the contrary. Alcoholism has increased in Japan, Korea, and some Chinese societies as opium use has waned (Singer, 1974). In North America, Mexican and Papago peoples had alcohol long before Euro-Americans arrived on the scene; but these groups have nonetheless had relatively high prevalence rates of alcoholism (Waddell, 1971).

Reasons for drinking can change over time, and they can be associated with psychiatric symptoms and disorder. For example, in traditional Latin American societies, drinking was largely a public and ceremonial or ritual behavior (Bunzel, 1940). However, individualistic "drinking to forget" has been found among Hispanic Americans in California. This particular motivation for drinking is associated with depression among Mexican American alcoholics (Goulding, Burnam, Benjamin, & Wells, 1993).

Communal Access to and Availability of Particular Psychoactive Substances

If a psychoactive substance is both nearby (i.e., available) and can be readily obtained (i.e., accessible), it is prone to use and abuse, especially if the group has no effective strictures against its use (Westermeyer, 1979). Three factors can enhance access of psychoactive substances in a community:

- production of a licit or illicit substance in the local community (e.g., tobacco in rural southeastern United States, scotch whiskey in Scotland, wine in France, opium in the Golden Triangle of Southeast Asia and the Golden Crescent of South Asia, cocaine in areas of South America, cannabis in the Caribbean, betel nut in South Asia);

- transportation and commerce through a non-producing commercial center (e.g., opium and later heroin in Hong Kong and Singapore, heroin and cocaine in Harlem, cocaine and cannabis in Miami and other ports of entry);

- active retail marketing of the substance, so that local inhabitants know where and when and how to obtain the substance.

A psychoactive substance can be available in a community, but not accessible to all inhabitants. This can be due to legal constraints: for example, minors cannot legally purchase certain licit psychoactive compounds. Certain prescribed substances can only be obtained with a physician's prescription. Cost can be a constraint, so that an expensive substance can only be purchased by those who can afford it. Ethnic affiliation can be a factor. For example, many Hmong refugees in the United States can obtain opium and many Ethiopian or Somali immigrants and refugees can obtain the plant stimulant qat, although most Americans have no notion of how to obtain these compounds (Westermeyer, Lyfoung, & Neider, 1989). Access and availability can change dramatically over time.

Much as ensocialization, access and availability can affect the rates of PSUD in a community, as well as the rates of PSUD-caused CMI (e.g., cocaine-precipitated psychoses), and rates of PSUD occurring in those with CMI (e.g., development of cannabis abuse in those with schizophrenia).

Psychoactive Substance as Cultural/Ethnic Symbol

Substances can achieve ethnic or cultural symbolism within and across cultures. This often occurs in a context of a multi-ethnic society or in a context of adjacent cultures that have widespread interaction *and* a need or wish to distinguish themselves from one another. For example, in India two groups maintain their separate identities, at least in part, through the exclusive use of either *daru* (an alcohol-containing beverage) or *bhang* (a cannabis compound) (Carstairs, 1954).

The same substance, used in different forms or in different ways, can also serve as a cultural symbol. For example, North Americans of para-Mediterranean heritage tend to drink wine during mealtimes at home during family rituals. In contrast, North Americans of Northern European heritage — at least during early generations following immigration — tended to drink beer or distilled beverages away from home among peers in ethnic bars or taverns (Bennett & Ames, 1985). The latter pattern of use tends to carry the risk of psychiatric maladies associated with episodic, heavy drinking.

Substances can also serve an a symbol of anti-governmental or anti-"social mainstream" attitudes. For example, the Irish during English colonial times distilled an illicit beverage alcohol called *poteen*. Likewise, American Indians continued to drink surreptitiously from the early 1800's to 1954 despite its being illegal for them to do so. Following the United States Narcotic Act of 1914, abuse of opiates, cannabis and cocaine largely disappeared from middle class Euro-Americans. However, abuse of these substances continued in urban pockets of African and Hispanic Americans (Bourgois, 1989). Illicit use of opiates among minority groups continued despite anti-opium laws in many countries of Asia (Westermeyer, 1983). Problems associated with this symbolic production and use of an illicit substance include the following: criminality, with its exposure to criminals and other criminal activities; rapid, surreptitious use to avoid detection, with its pathogenic properties; and use outside of the ethnic mainstream, so that non-ritual, non-family use patterns are fostered. Even when adverse political or economic circumstances change, the ethnic group may continue its use of the illicit substance, as exemplified by the continued distillation of *poteen* in Ireland even after independence from England.

Some substances may possess sacramental status in certain ethnic groups. For example, the hallucinogen peyote is a sacramental intoxicant that is key to the religious experience in the Native

American Church. Although adherents of that religion treat the substance with great respect and do not abuse it, non-believers with access to the substance may abuse it, with subsequent psychiatric complications. Similarly, wine is a sacramental in the Catholic Church, a faith with origins in the Mediterranean. Although para-Mediterranean clergy experience little or no problems with this sacramental, sacramental wine abuse has been so frequent among clergy of northern European origins that asylum and treatment facilities for alcoholic clergy have been established in North America and elsewhere.

Consuming the same intoxicant in the same setting can serve as a means for integrating disparate ethnic groups. For example, taverns in South America and Africa have been places for meeting and discussion among people of different ethnic affiliations. Despite their obvious function of bringing people together in a fairly egalitarian fashion, such taverns also foster a non-family, peer-oriented style of drinking, with its risk for alcoholism.

An extreme example of a strongly pathogenic use pattern as practiced by certain plains and woodland Indian tribal groups, are characterized by the following:

• learning to drink among slightly older peers in a surreptitious fashion;

• drinking over a period of days, at times until all financial resources are exhausted;

• drinking together with a group, which moves or travels even after bars close;

• refusal to drink with the group in the way that the group drinks is considered an insult or "acting better than we are";

• placing other priorities, such as work or family obligations, behind the drinking activity.

Psychoactive Substance as Economic Resource

Production, transportation and sale of licit and illicit psychoactive substances comprises a major industry in many areas of the world. Insofar as the producers are middle class members of the ethnic majority, the substance and its associated commercial activities tend to be licit. Examples include Scots-English landholders, businessmen, and corporate executives involved in the tobacco industry of southeastern United States. The whiskey industry in Kentucky-Tennessee is a similar example, as is the German beer producing industry in several areas around the United States and the Italian-Spanish wine industry of the western and southwestern United States.

On the other hand, poorer ethnic groups outside of the socioeconomic "mainstream" have tended to engage in illicit production, transport and sale of psychoactive substances. Examples have included Sicilian-Italians and Corsican-French in heroin commerce, Hispanic Americans and African Americans in heroin and cocaine commerce, and Hmong refugees in opium commerce (Bourgois, 1989; Westermeyer, 1983). Formerly "mainstream" farmers and chemists in the United States have become involved with illicit production of cannabis and "designer drugs" as they have encountered economic reversals. It seems likely that economic factors operate strongly in these social trends, perhaps bolstered by frustration at being unable to become part of the economic "mainstream" of the society. Absence of an ethnic taboo against the activity no doubt plays a role as well. For this reason, ethnic minorities who abuse illicit drugs, such as heroin and cocaine, appear to be more psychologically "normal" on various psychological measures than ethnic "mainstream" drug abusers (Craig & Baker, 1982). However, these differences on psychological tests do not hold in some studies of clinical populations. For example, Kosten, Rounsaville, and Kleber (1985) observed more schizophrenia, anxiety disorders, and depressive symptoms among 60 Puerto Rican opiate addicts as compared to males of other ethnic groups. Of interest, they found more antisocial personality among 177 White male addicts as compared to the other ethnic groups, suggesting that these ethnic "mainstream" patients were more sociopathic in order to undertake a behavior that was more taboo in their racial group.

These demographic aspects of illicit drug commerce have certain implications for persons with PSUD and CMI. One consequence is the tendency within communities for producers and traffickers in a substance to become users and, eventually, abusers of the substance (Westermeyer, 1983). Widespread PSUD in these communities both precipitates and complicates CMI. Traumatic brain injury associated with criminality and "gang warfare" over drug commerce "rights" is another cause of associated PSUD-CMI (Bourgois, 1989).

Male Versus Female Rates of PSUD and CMI

Overall, PSUD tends to occur more commonly among men than women. There are certain exceptions, however. For example, sedative abuse in the United States and Canada has tended to occur more frequently among women than men (Ross, 1989). The proportion of women dependent on tobacco in the United States is rapidly approaching the rate among men. Despite these exceptions, the rate of PSUD among men tends to exceed that among women. Given equal cross-sex access to any given substance, the ratio of men-to-women with PSUD ranges around two or three men to one woman. This is true with a variety of substances, including alcohol and opiates, and in a diversity of ethnic groups (Arif & Westermeyer, 1988; Westermeyer, 1980-b; Westermeyer, 1993). Thus, one would anticipate, based on this statistic alone, that PSUD and CMI would accompany one another more often among men than among women. Of course, this would not be true if other factors were operating to "immunize" persons with PSUD against CMI; however, in general the opposite appears to be the case.

Cultural and ethnic examples do occur in which the gender ratio falls well above the usual two or three men to one woman. One example is Hispanic Americans, among whom male alcoholism is relatively common but female alcoholism is relatively infrequent (Fernandez-Pol, Bluestone, Morales, & Mizrucki, 1985). The same appears to be true for heroin dependence among Hispanic Americans (Almog, Anglin, & Fisher, 1993). Several factors appear to account for this, such as:

- alcohol intoxication, especially in public, is acceptable for men in many South American cultures, but not for women;

- women's role vis-a-vis male drunkenness is to rescue the man and control or protect him during his vulnerability while intoxicated;

- the "macho" role condones drinking whereas the "mariana" role supports sober and maternal caring;

- strong cultural taboos and loss of status follow upon female intoxication and female participation in peer-group drinking.

Opiate addiction in Asia evidences vastly different gender ratios. For example, the usual two-to-three males to one female addict predominates among ethnic/cultural groups engaged in the production of opium poppy (Westermeyer, 1980-b). In most of these groups, women play an active role in poppy culture and opium harvesting: opium is available in the home, where it is often used as a medicament or a social intoxicant by these groups (with the notable exception of the Turks). Among ethnic/cultural groups engaged in opium commerce, however, the proportion of women addicts is considerably less. In these latter societies, men are exposed to opium through their roles as merchants, muleteers, boatmen, truck drivers, policemen and bankers. They may also frequent opium dens, where the clientele is predominantly male. Women are not introduced to opium through their work or social roles, unless their husband brings it into the home or they are engaged in an occupation that involves opium use (e.g., prostitution) (Bourgois, 1989; Westermeyer, 1974-b). In most settings, the gender ratio of men-to-women tends to be greater with illicit drugs (i.e., more men) and smaller with licit drugs (i.e., more women) (Sutker, Archer, & Allain, 1980; Westermeyer, 1980-b). This suggests that women tend to be more sensitive to and compliant with socio-legal taboos than do men. This potential psychocultural characteristic could of course be associated with lower rates of certain CMI (e.g., antisocial personality disorder) but could theoretically be associated with higher rates of other CMI (e.g., mood disorder, obsessive compulsive disorder). Existence of gender-related PSUD-CMI comorbidities is supported by some research findings (Kosten et al., 1985).

ETHNIC/CULTURAL VARIABILITY IN ACCESS TO AND EFFECTIVENESS OF TREATMENT

Ethnicity has been observed to affect access to PSUD treatment over the last few decades, a factor which may be related to CMI. For example, a treatment program in the middle of New York City was observed to attract Euro-Americans and Blacks in large numbers, but did not attract Hispanic Americans despite their large numbers of PSUD problems and their proximity to the treatment facility (Kane, 1981). Opium treatment facilities in Asia have also been observed to attract different patient populations based on age, race, religion, language, and sex (Westermeyer, 1980-a). These data suggest that individuals with PSUD do not readily present themselves to treatment facilities that they perceive as not serving their ethnic group. This can occur despite the availability of the treatment resource in the community, or the absence of socioeconomic barriers to the treatment resource. Quasi-experimental reports have indicated that this "lack of access" can be easily reversed by simply hiring people who share ethnic identity and affiliation with the target population that does not see the facility as accessible (Westermeyer, Tanner, & Smelker, 1976).

Even in the presence of availability and access to treatment, differences may exist in the efficacy of treatment across ethnic/cultural boundaries. For example, we observed that 100 American Indian patients with PSUD had the same access as other patients with PSUD to both treatment for PSUD *and* treatment for psychiatric disorder (Westermeyer, in press). However, the Native American patients had much higher rates of psychiatric diagnoses overall than the other patients. Since many (but not all) of these diagnoses were related to chronic PSUD, especially chronic alcoholism, lack of treatment efficacy for PSUD could be a pathogenic factor in the adverse course manifested by the American Indian patients. Another possibility is that lack of efficacy of treatment for psychiatric disorders might have been conducive to PSUD, since a higher-than-expected number of American Indian patients had an anxiety disorder associated with their PSUD. Other data support these findings of a poor prognosis for American Indian alcoholics (Westermeyer & Peake, 1983) as compared to a good prognosis overall for treated alcoholics in the United States and Canada (Smart & Mann, 1993).

Prognosis with alcohol-related liver disease differs among ethnic groups in the United States, suggesting different treatment courses for alcoholism as a function of ethnicity. Mendenhall, Gartside, Roselle, Grossman, Weesner, and Chedid (1989) found the following survival rates for alcohol-related liver disease at 42 months: African Americans 66%, Caucasian Americans 40%, Hispanic Americans 28%, American Indians 0%.

Keene and Raynor (1993) have observed the congruence/incongruence of client/therapist beliefs in a sample of English people with alcoholism treated in an A.A.-oriented program. They found that longer stay and compliance with treatment were related to similarity in beliefs regarding the client's problems and their clinical management. This may extend to other ethnic/cultural beliefs related to concepts regarding health-illness, treatment and recovery.

Access to and utilization of mental health services also differ across ethnicities. In particular, Mexican Americans tend to use such services less than do other ethnic groups (Briones, Heller, Chalfant, Roberts, Aguirre-Hauchbaum, & Farr, 1990). Factors contributing to this phenomenon appear to include socioeconomic status, degree of acculturation, world views such as fatalism, and focus on the family and the individual as exclusive sources of help in the face of personal crisis. This may foster the use of substances for self therapy of CMI, as described elsewhere in this chapter.

CONCLUSIONS AND COMMENTS

In the relative absence of definitive studies of cultural and ethnic influences on substance abuse among persons with severe mental illness, the following statements can be offered as plausible hypotheses.

1. Ethnic and cultural groups may *differ in their rates of PSUD and PSUD-related CMI* as a result of the following:

- *Type* of psychoactive substance *and pattern of use* that are prescribed, approved or permitted by the group;

- *Behavioral norms* in the group regarding types of psychoactive substances and approved patterns of use;

- *Availability* of psychoactive substances in the community (i.e., presence of substance in the environment);

- *Access* of people in the community to the psychoactive substance (i.e., they know where and how to obtain it and have the resources to do so);

- *Symbolic meaning* of the substance in the group, as related to the group's identity, their world view, and their values.

- *Economic role* of the substance to the group: does the substance generate subsistence income or possible wealth for the group or individuals within the group?

2. *Ensocialization* of children, adolescents and young adults can *protect* against PSUD and PSUD-related CMI. Means by which this can be accomplished include:

- Teaching children to consume psychoactive substances for social or recreation purposes only on *socially sanctioned, ritual or ceremonial, multigenerational occasions when food is served;*

- *No individual use* of taboo or proscribed psychoactive substances (an exception is medically controlled administration for licit health reasons).

3. *Ensocialization* may *fail* to protect against PSUD and PSUD-related CMI if:

- The person *leaves the group-of-origin* for life in an adopted group;

- The person uses a psychoactive substance for which *no prescription or proscription* has been provided by the ensocializing group;

- The values instilled by the group-of-origin are *overcome by other values* of another group or culture (e.g., "youth culture," secular culture);

- *Conflict* between *ideal* and *behavioral norms* (i.e., the group is supposed to be abstinent from the substance, but some people decide to use the substance anyway).

4. *Men* and *women* may *differ* across ethnic groups and cultures in their rates of PSUD and PSUD-related CMI as a consequence of the following:

- *Men* tend to have *higher rates* of PSUD for most substances as compared to women in virtually all known groups, but the sex ratio can differ from one group to the next in association with sex-related differences in values and access (e.g., "marianisma" among Latin American women);

- *Men* are more apt to consume socially unapproved or *illicit* psychoactive substances as compared to women.

5. *Treatment access and efficacy* for PSUD and for CMI can differ across ethnic and cultural groups. This can affect the prevalence of the disorder (i.e., the rate that is usually studied in PSUD and CMI) even though the incidence might be the same in the two societies (since incidence is rarely studied in psychiatric conditions). Delayed treatment or ineffective treatment for PSUD may contribute to comorbid CMI.

REFERENCES

Almog, Y. J., Anglin, M. D., & Fisher, D. G. (1993). Alcohol and heroin use patterns of narcotics addicts: Gender and ethnic differences. *American Journal of Drug and Alcohol Abuse, 19*(2), 219–238.

Arif, A., & Westermeyer, J. (Ed.). (1988). *A Manual for Drug and Alcohol Abuse.* New York: Praeger.

Bauman, K. E., Foshee, V. A., Linzer, M. A., & Koch, G. G. (1990). Effect of parental smoking classification on the association between parental and adolescent smoking. *Addictive Behaviors, 15,* 413–422.

Bennett, L. A., & Ames, G. M. (Ed.). (1985). *The American Experience With Alcohol: Contrasting Cultural Perspectives.* New York: Plenum Press.

Bourgois, P. (1989). In search of Horatio Alger: Culture and ideology in the crack community. *Contemporary Drug Problems,* Winter, 619–649.

Brady, M. (1990). Indigenous and government attempts to control alcohol use among Australian Aborigines. *Contemporary Drug Problems, Summer,* 195–220.

Bunzel, R. (1940). The role of alcoholism in two Central American cultures. *Psychiatry, 3,* 361–387.

Carpenter, M. A., & Ewing, J. A. (1989). The outbreeding of alcoholism. *American Journal Drug Alcohol Abuse, 15*(1), 93–99.

Carstairs, G. M. (1954). Daru and bhang: Cultural factors in the choice of intoxicant. *Quarterly Journal of Studies on Alcohol, 15,* 220–237.

Craig, R. J., & Baker, S. (Ed.). (1982). *Drug Dependent Patients: Treatment and Research.* Springfield, IL: Charles C. Thomas.

Eaton, J., & Weil, R. (1955). *Culture and Mental Disorder.* Glencoe,IL: Free Press.

Fernandez-Pol, B., Bluestone, H., Morales, G., & Mizrucki, M. (1985). Cultural influences and alcoholism: A study of Puerto Ricans. *Alcoholism:Clinical and Experimental Research, 9*(5), 443–446.

Gfroerer, J., & DeLaRosa, M. (1993). Protective and risk factors associated with drug use among Hispanic Youth. *Journal of Addictive Diseases, 12*(2), 87–107.

Giacopassi, D. J., & Stein, P. M. (1991). The intoxication power of alcoholic beverages: Image and reality. *American Journal of Drug and Alcohol Abuse, 17*(4), 429–438.

Goulding, J. M., Burnam, M. A., Benjamin, B., & Wells, K. B. (1993). Risk factors for secondary depression among Mexican Americans and Non-Hispanic Whites: Alcohol use, alcohol dependence, and reasons for drinking. *Journal of Nervous and Mental Disease, 181*(3), 166–175.

Isreal, Y., Orrego, H., Schmidt, W., Popham, R. E., Escartin, P., Ishii, H., Kelly, D., Long, J. P., Malizia, G., Mezey, E., Pagliaro, T., Salaspuro, M., & Tanikawa, K. (1991). Trauma in cirrhosis: An indicator of the pattern of alcohol abuse in different societies. *Alcohol: Clinical and Experimental Research, 15*(3), 433–437.

Kane, G. (1981). *Inner City Alcoholism: An Ecological and Cross-Cultural Study.* New York: Human Science Press.

Keaulana, K. A., & Whitney, S. (1990). Ka wai kau mai o Maleka "Water from America": the intoxication of the Hawai'ian people. *Contemporary Drug Problems,* Summer, 161–194.

Keene, J., & Raynor, P. (1993). Addiction as a 'soul sickness': The influence of client and therapist beliefs. *Addiction Research, 1,* 77–87.

Kosten, T. R., Rounsaville, B. J., & Kleber, H. D. (1985). Ethnic and gender differences among opiate addicts. *Internatlional Journal of Addictions, 20*(8), 1143–1162.

Lee, C. K., Kwak, Y. S., Yamamoto, J., Rhee, H., Kim, Y. S., Han, J. H., Choi, J. O., & Lee, Y. H. (1990). Psychiatric epidemiology in Korea; Part I: Gender and age differences in Seoul. *Journal of Nervous and Mental Disease, 178*(4), 242–246.

MacAndrew, C., & Edgerton, R. B. (1969). *Drunken Comportment: A Social Explanation.* Chicago: Aldine.

Maddahian, E., Newcomb, M. D., & Bentler, P. M. (1986). Adolescents' substance use: Impact of ethnicity, income, and availability. *Advances in Alcohol and Substance Abuse, 5*(3), 63–79.

Mendenhall, C. L., Gartside, P. S., Roselle, G. A., Grossman, C. J., Weesner, R. E., & Chedid, A. (1989). Longevity among ethnic groups in alcoholic liver disease. *Alcohol and Alcoholism, 24*(1), 11–19.

Padilla, E. R., Padilla, A. M., Ramirea, R., Morales, A., & Olmedo, E.L. (1977). *Inhalant, Marijuana and Alcohol Abuse among Barrio Children and Adolescemts.* Los Angeles: University of California Spanish Speaking Mental Health Research Center.

Ringwalt, C. L., & Palmer, J. H. (1990). Differences between White and Black youth who drink heavily. *Addictive Behaviors, 15,* 455–460.

Roberts, B. H., & Myers, J. K. (1967). Religion, national origin, immigration, and mental illness. In S. K. Weinberg (Eds.), *The Sociology of Mental Disorders* Chicago: Aldine.

Ross, H. E. (1989). Alcohol and drug abuse in treated alcoholics: A comparison of men and women. *Alcoholism: Clinical and Experimental Research, 13*(6), 810–816.

Singer, K. (1974). The choice of intoxicant among the Chinese. *British Journal of Addiction, 69,* 257–258.

Smart, R. E., & Mann, R. E. (1993). Recent liver cirrhosis declines: estimates of the impact of alcohol abuse treatment and alcoholics anonymous. *Addiction, 88*, 193–198.

Sutker, P. B., Archer, R. P., & Allain, A. N. (1980). Psychopathology of drug abusers: Sex and ethnic considerations. *International Journal of Addictions, 15*, 605–613.

Teck-Hong, O. (1986). Inhalant abuse in Singapore. *International Journal of Addictions, 21*(8), 955–960.

Waddell, J. O. (1971). "Drink friend!": Social context of convivial drinking and drunkenness among Papagos in an urban setting. In *Proceedings of the First Annual Alcoholism Conference of NIAAA,* E. Chafetz (Ed.). Washington, DC: U.S. Printing Office.

Westermeyer, J. (1974-a). 'The drunken Indian': Myths and realities. *Psychiatric Annals, 4*, 29–35.

Westermeyer, J. (1974-b). Opium dens: A social resource for addicts in Laos. *Archives of General Psychiatry, 31*, 237–240.

Westermeyer, J. (1979). Influence of opium availability on addiction rates in Laos. *American Journal of Epidemiology, 109*, 550–562.

Westermeyer, J. (1980-a). Medical and nonmedical treatment for narcotic addicts: A comparative study from Asia. *Journal of Nervous and Mental Disease, 167*, 205–211.

Westermeyer, J. (1980-b). Sex ratio among opium addicts in Asia: Influences of drug availability and sampling method. *Drug Alcohol Dependence, 6*, 131–136.

Westermeyer, J. (1983). *Poppies, Pipes and People: Opium and Its Use in Laos.* Berkeley, California: University of California Press.

Westermeyer, J. (1993). Psychiatric disorder among American Indian versus other patients with Psychoactive Substance Use Disorder. *American Journal of Addictions. 2*, 309–314.

Westermeyer, J., Lyfoung, T., & Neider, J. (1989). An epidemic of opium dependence among Asian refugees in the U.S.: Characteristics and causes. *British Journal of Addiction, 84*, 785–789.

Westermeyer, J., & Peake, E. (1983). A ten year follow up of alcoholic Native Americans in Minnesota. *American Journal of Psychiatry, 140*, 189–194.

Westermeyer, U., Tanner, R., & Smelker, J. (1976). Staff integration at a neighborhood health center. *Urban Health, 5*, 43–48.

Wingert, J. L., & Fifield, M. G. (1985). Characteristics of Native American users of inhalants. *International Journal of Addictions, 20*(10), 1575–1582.

4

Assessment of Substance Use Among Persons with Chronic Mental Illnesses

ROBERT E. DRAKE and CAROLYN MERCER-MCFADDEN

INTRODUCTION

This chapter reviews procedures for identifying and evaluating substance use among individuals with severe mental illness (SMI). The approach to assessment described here stems from the biopsychosocial model of addiction and is consistent with current knowledge regarding the comprehensive treatment of persons with dual disorders. Assessment is both an ongoing process and a therapeutic intervention in itself. Depending on the client's level of engagement, awareness, motivation, capacity, and resources, the assessment process serves to educate and involve the client and significant others in treatment.

According to the biopsychosocial model, the manifest behaviors related to substance use are multidimensional phenomena that are developed and maintained by multiple, interacting factors (Donovan, 1988). Consequently, approaches to assessment, to treatment planning, and to treatment itself must simultaneously address several critical variables — from biological, psychological, and social spheres. The biopsychosocial model gives the assessment process an expanded role in treatment because treatment is highly individualized and completely dependent on the ongoing, dynamic assessment process (Lehman, Myers & Corty, 1989). Moreover, because knowledge about causation, course, and treatment is evolving rapidly, assessment will continue to be refined in the next several years. This approach to assessment, based on empirical hypothesis testing of clinical diagnosis and treatment, is consistent with current knowledge regarding the comprehensive treatment of dual disorders (Drake, Bartels, Teague, Noordsy, & Clark, 1993-b).

Assessment incorporates several functions: identifying problems, bringing them into clear focus, establishing working diagnoses, forming a relationship, helping to motivate the client, negotiating a contract, and setting the stage for an intervention (Kofoed, 1991). Assessment includes four stages — detection, classification, specialized assessment, and treatment planning — and merges with treatment. The stages overlap in time; each typically results in feedback and revisions of the results of previously completed procedures (see Figure 4.1).

Detection procedures focus on identifying substance dependence, substance abuse, or harmful or dangerous use that does not qualify for a diagnosis (Babor, Kranzler & Lauerman, 1989). The products of detection are: 1) identification of problem areas, and 2) determination of further classification and assessment procedures to be used.

Classification procedures evaluate the DSM-III-R diagnosis of substance use disorder and the comorbid psychiatric disorder. Classification of substance use in persons with SMI is problematic because the usual criteria for determining nonproblematic use, for assessing quantity and frequency of use, for identifying typical consequences, and for the dependence syndrome may be different for persons with SMI than for others. Classification produces a description of the clinical phenomena under study, a clinical understanding of the symptom pattern, hypotheses for further specialized assessment — including hypotheses about DSM-III-R diagnoses — and choice of general types of treatment interventions.

Specialized assessment procedures entail a more thorough analysis of the substance-related problems, including the severity of disorder and stage of treatment, and of the biopsychosocial factors that ap-

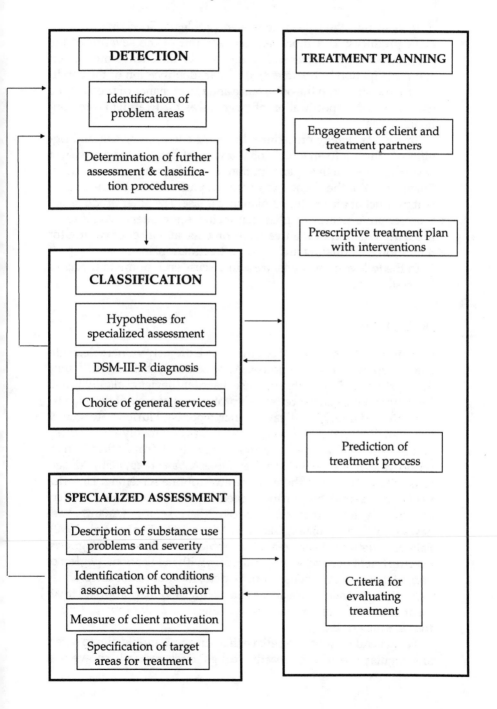

pear to sustain the substance-related problems. Specialized assessment produces: 1) a more detailed account of the severity of the substance-related problems; 2) a measure of the client's motivation and participation in treatment; 3) a clear identification of the conditions associated with the occurrence and maintenance of problematic use, and; 4) the specification of target areas for treatment interventions.

Treatment planning procedures bring the client, clinicians, and significant others into an educational review of data for the purpose of ensuring their active participation in appropriate interventions. Engagement of the client and treatment partners can be one important product of the treatment planning phase. The other products are a prescriptive treatment plan that includes the interventions to be tried, a prediction of the treatment process, and a set of criteria for monitoring, evaluating and revising treatment plans.

In the following sections, we will discuss each of the four phases in greater detail.

DETECTION

Psychiatric clients with SMI constitute an extremely vulnerable, high-risk group for substance abuse. Approximately half meet lifetime diagnostic criteria for substance use disorder (Regier et al., 1990), and even more have substance-related problems that are not detected by standardized interview (Drake, Osher, Noordsy, Hurlbutt, Teague, & Beaudett, 1990). Although alcohol is the most commonly abused drug, persons with SMI are prone to abuse a variety of drugs other than alcohol (Mueser et al., 1990; Sevy, Kay, Opler & Van Praag, 1990). All persons with SMI should therefore receive routine screening. Unfortunately, only a small proportion of clients with substance use disorders are typically detected in acute care psychiatric settings (Ananth, Vandewater, Kamal, Broksky, Gamal & Miller, 1989; Drake et al., 1990). Failure to detect substance-related problems results in misdiagnosis; overtreatment of psychiatric syndromes with medications; neglect of appropriate interventions such as detoxification, substance abuse education, and substance abuse counseling; and inappropriate treatment planning and referral (Drake, Alterman & Rosenberg, 1993-a; Ries & Samson, 1987).

For several reasons, we believe that screening should aim to detect any regular use of psychoactive drugs. First, research shows that attempts at controlled use of psychoactive substances in persons with SMI are highly likely to result in substance use disorder over time (Drake and Wallach, 1994). Second, probably due to biological vulnerability, even small amounts of alcohol (Drake, Osher, & Wallach, 1989) or other drugs (Lieberman, Kinon & Loebel, 1990) are associated with negative outcomes for this population. Third, persons with SMI are often unaware of or confused about the consequences of their substance use, and any report of regular use is likely to signify disorder (Dixon, DiBietz, Myers, Conley, Medoff & Lehman, 1993).

Although the lack of screening instruments and procedures to detect alcohol and drug-related problems in persons with SMI is a critical part of the problem, a few simple procedures could dramatically improve current rates of detection (Drake et al., 1993-a).

Laboratory Tests

Urine drug testing is probably the most feasible and effective approach currently available for detecting illicit drug use in persons with SMI. These tests provide only limited information on quantity and frequency, and negative tests can be attributed to many sources other than abstinence (Gold & Dackis, 1986). Nevertheless, positive tests, particularly with repeated urine testing, are common in persons with SMI (Blumberg, Cohen, Heaton, & Klein, 1971), even among clients who deny use and are not suspected of abuse by their clinicians (Stone, Greenstein, Gable & McClellan, 1993). Routine urine drug screening is often recommended for all incoming psychiatric clients (Safer, 1987). We also recommend repeated testing for all clients in high-risk categories (such as those with frequent relapses, aggressive outbursts, or unstable housing) and for those returning to inpatient care after community visits (Drake et al., 1993-a).

Blood and urine tests for alcohol are not as helpful as urine testing for other drugs because alcohol is metabolized and excreted rapidly. Even indirect tests, such as liver enzymes and red blood cell morphology, are primarily sensitive to heavy alcohol use in the past few weeks (Babor, et al., 1989). Breathalyzer assessments, though sensitive for only a few hours or less, are more convenient and less costly. While they have not been studied in the SMI population, we recommend using breathalyzers in high-risk situations, e.g., at the time of inpatient admission or emergency room visit (Drake et al., 1993-a).

Self-Report

Direct interview and questionnaires are validly used to detect substance use disorders (Babor, Stephen & Marlatt, 1987). Both approaches can be problematic in acute treatment settings for a variety of reasons, including noncompliance, minimization, and distortion due to cognitive impairment or psychosis, and researchers have documented significant underreporting of drug abuse in persons with SMI (Mueser et al., 1990; Stone et al., 1993). Nevertheless, self-reported information about substance use can be helpful when clients are willing to acknowledge their use. We recommend using a short self-report instrument to document the frequency of use of alcohol, of all major classes of illicit drugs, and of non-prescribed medications over the past 30 days and over some longer interval (Drake et al., 1993-a). Several conditions probably increase the validity of self-report: the client is psychiatrically stable; the interview is careful, nonjudgmental, and confidential; and the information is collected in conjunction with laboratory assessment. For those in high-risk categories, assessments should be repeated regularly (e.g., every month).

Psychiatric clients may be more willing to acknowledge alcohol use than illicit drug use. They are also more able to report frequency of alcohol use than to identify consequences of alcohol use. For the reasons cited above, any use of alcohol should be assessed carefully. Standard questionnaires and interviews can be used successfully with this population, although lengthy interviews may not be practical in acute care situations (Barbee, Clark, Crapanzano, Heintz & Kehoe, 1989). Questions that refer to complaints about drinking by family members (McHugo, Paskus & Drake, 1993) or to regular use (Dixon et al., 1993) may be the most pertinent.

Physical Signs and Symptoms

Several signs and symptoms such as pupillary changes and rapid heart rate are consistent with the effects of specific drugs, but these indicators overlap considerably with the signs of various psychotic and agitated states. Nevertheless, treatment staff and other observers are frequently quite sensitive to the effects of alcohol and other drugs, and trained case managers, who observe clients regularly in the community, may be the best single source of detection (Drake et al., 1990; Test, Wallish, Allness & Ripp, 1989). The role of medical history and medical exam for this population are unclear at this point.

Collateral Sources

The case managers' sensitivity to detection may stem from their close contact with family and other collaterals. Although friends and other informants may have incomplete information and many persons with SMI are socially isolated, close personal contacts, such as family, friends, and housing staff, can be helpful in identifying substance abuse. Since alcohol use is legal and often more public, collateral informants may be more aware of alcohol use than illicit drug use.

Correlates

Some of the typical clinical correlates of substance abuse, such as marital difficulties, smoking cigarettes, and job problems, are not particularly helpful in detecting substance abuse among persons with SMI. Several studies (Alterman, Erdlen, McLellan, & Mann, 1980; Alterman, Erdlen, LaPorte & Erdlen, 1982; Dixon, Haas, Weiden, Sweeney & Frances, 1990; Drake & Wallach, 1989; Drake, Wallach, Teague, Freeman, Paskus & Clark, 1991-a; Mueser et al., 1990) indicate that other correlates are important: family history, youth, male gender, unstable housing, homelessness, disruptive behavior, treatment noncompliance, legal difficulties, incarceration, frequent relapses, and friends who are antisocial or drug abusers. The presence of one or more of these correlates should alert the clinician to a high index of suspicion.

CLASSIFICATION

Diagnosis, though subtle and fraught with problems of validity in persons with SMI, probably has several roles beyond serving as a trigger for reimbursements. The current interest in diagnosing substance use disorder in psychiatric settings may increase its salience, improve the prospects for detection, enhance the potential for treatment, and induce more of a demand for training among clinicians.

Applying DSM-III-R criteria for psychoactive substance use disorders to the SMI population is admittedly difficult. The criteria for what constitutes abuse and dependence have been established and validated largely in persons with single disorders or with less severe psychopathology, and these criteria may not be clinically significant in the context of co-occurring SMI. For example, these clients may be so vulnerable that they encounter difficulties with small amounts of substance use before they acquire the dependence syndrome (Drake et al., 1990). In addition, the typical consequences of substance abuse are different for persons with SMI, e.g., medication noncompliance, unstable housing, and rehospitalization. Perhaps the most difficult problem is sorting out the consequences of substance use, mental disorder, and medication non-compliance when the three co-occur (Drake et al., 1989). Nonetheless, longitudinal observation should allow clinicians and clients to recognize if substance use meets the DSM-III-R criterion of causing persistent dysfunction in social, vocational, psychological, or physical functioning.

Several authors have discussed the difficulties of establishing diagnoses in the context of mixed substance use and symptoms of severe mental illness (Dixon et al., 1993; Kofoed, 1991; Lehman et al., 1989; Lehman, Myers, Corty & Thompson, in press; Osher & Kofoed, 1989; Rosenthal, Hellerstein and Miner, 1992; Weiss, Mirin, & Griffin, 1992). Consensus exists at least on the necessity of using a longitudinal, open-ended process. Most researchers also agree that the primary-secondary distinction is problematic, especially when the distinction is based on temporal course, and that this distinction usually does not help in making clinical decisions. Therefore, severe mental disorder and substance use disorder should, in most cases, be identified as two separate diagnoses. Finally, most researchers also agree that diagnosing substance use disorder is more straightforward than diagnosing other psychiatric diagnoses among persons with SMI. We will discuss the two issues separately.

Diagnosis of Comorbid Substance Use Disorder

Substance use disorder can be diagnosed reliably early in the assessment process (Kofoed, 1991). The key criterion, as mentioned above, is the persistence of adverse social, psychological, vocational, or medical consequences related to substance use. The clinician should remember that clients with SMI are extremely vulnerable to the effects of psychoactive substances, that the consequences they suffer may be different from the usual consequences in persons without a concurrent mental illness, and that clients are likely to be confused about or unaware of consequences. Any regular use of alcohol or other drugs should be considered potentially harmful use and will indicate disorder in a high proportion of individuals (Dixon, et al., 1993).

Although structured interviews probably yield the best data, they may miss 25% of those abusing alcohol, even in optimal circumstances (Drake et al., 1990). Interviews may miss an even higher proportion of those abusing illicit substances (Stone et al., 1993). A brief interview may be as accurate as a lengthy interview (McHugo et al., 1993). As noted above, the best approach may entail longitudinal observations of use and consequences, multiple perspectives, laboratory tests, and a high level of suspicion.

Diagnosis of Comorbid Psychiatric Disorder

Little consensus exists on the method, timing, and choice of psychiatric diagnoses to make in the context of substance use disorder. Most structured interviews use exclusion questions regarding whether, for example, symptoms always occur in relation to substance use, and most clinicians recommend conducting interviews after a period of abstinence. Nevertheless, problems remain regarding the necessary length of abstinence, the client's confusion, and the boundaries between organically induced symptoms and symptoms of an autonomous disorder. Lehman et al. (1994) and Rosenthal et al. (1992) have documented the high proportion of cases in which the psychiatric disorder cannot be clearly classified as independent of the substance use disorder or dependent upon it.

Weiss and colleagues (1992) have recently made the following set of recommendations: Use a longitudinal evaluation process and multiple sources of data; delay interviews until the client is psychiatrically and physically stable, and use clinically trained interviewers who understand the specific short- and long-term effects of each individual drug of abuse. To these recommendations Kofoed (1991) adds the caveat that the psychiatric presentation is likely to change with prolonged abstinence, so psychiatric symptoms and diagnoses, as well as treatments, should be periodically reevaluated.

SPECIALIZED ASSESSMENT

Specialized assessment yields thorough and specific information for planning treatment. Substance use disorder is considered a complex behavior pattern with multiple, interacting components. Assessment procedures and the scope of the investigation are based on clinical hypotheses about DSM-III-R diagnoses generated in the detection and classification phases (Donovan, 1988). The client is continuously involved in developing hypotheses, reviewing clinical data, specifying strategies for further assessment, and planning interventions. Specialized assessment thoroughly explores three areas: the nature and severity of the problematic substance-using behaviors, the important conditions that are associated with the occurrence and maintenance of the problematic substance-using behaviors, and the target areas for intervention.

Nature and Severity of Substance-Using Behaviors

The substance-using behaviors should first be clearly and thoroughly described (Donovan, 1988). Description should address the time, duration, frequency, level of intensity, and quantity of use; the severity of the problem; the developmental history of use; the physiological, cognitive, behavioral, and environmental systems that are involved in the behaviors; and the immediate and delayed consequences of use. For example, physiological factors include family history, which may imply genetic vulnerability; tolerance, dependence, and withdrawal; and the medical sequelae of substance use. Cognitive factors include positive and negative expectancies related to use, such as enhanced mood, improved social ease, increased cognitive function, or enhanced feelings of arousal. Behavioral factors include interpersonal coping strategies and communication skills. Environmental factors include the social context of use, such as peer pressure.

Severity is determined in terms of the intensity, stereotypy, and autonomous character of the behavioral, cognitive, and physiological conditions associated with use of the substance (Donovan, 1988). Because substance use disorder is heterogeneous, assessment must investigate all of the relevant domains but be individualized and correspond to the duration of the substance-using behavior (Skinner, 1981). For example, extensive neuropsychological testing may not be important for the young, moderate drinker but is often critical for an older person with a long drinking history (Donovan, Kivlahan, Walker & Umlauf, 1985). For dually diagnosed persons, the usefulness of many assessment procedures remains to be determined.

Another important dimension of description is the individual's stage of change and stage of treatment. Prochaska, DiClemente, and Norcross (1992) have found that individuals with substance use disorder change in a predictable sequence, whether they do so on their own or in relation to a treatment program. They identify five stages of change: (1) *precontemplation*, in which the individual has little or no awareness of a problem and no intention to change; (2) *contemplation*, in which there is awareness of a problem and some consideration of change but no commitment to change; (3) *preparation*, which includes some, perhaps unsuccessful attempts to change and the intention to take further action; (4) *action*, during which the individual expends time and energy to effect behavioral changes; and (5) *maintenance*, which involves continued activity to prevent relapse and to consolidate changes.

Osher and Kofoed (1989) independently derived a parallel scheme for the stage of treatment. Their scheme includes the concept of a stage of change, consistent with the ideas of Prochaska and colleagues. They also include the concept of the client's level of involvement in the treatment program, adding the perspective of the provider who is actively attempting to help the client to change. A client in the *engagement* stage develops a trusting relationship with treatment staff, often one or more case managers. During *persuasion*, clients learn more about the role that alcohol and drugs have played in their lives and develop motivation for change. They use specific strategies and interventions during *active treatment* to reduce their substance use and to attain abstinence. When these gains are stable, other specific strategies are employed as part of *relapse prevention*.

Conditions Associated with Substance-Using Behaviors

A detailed description of the substance-using behaviors flows directly into an analysis of the associated conditions that appear to be involved in maintaining the disorder. Even the most severe addiction involves more than a physiological progression. Social learning interacts with physiological processes as they are interpreted, labeled, and given meaning by the individual (Lindesmith, 1968). Over time the interactions among physiological, cognitive, behavioral, and environmental components determine the individual's internal set and the external settings that maintain the behaviors (Zinberg, 1984). To understand the complex, individualized pattern of the constituent elements and how to intervene represents the exciting clinical challenge with each client.

Current assessment procedures may not be equal to the task. Standardized instruments do exist to address physiological processes, cognitive deficits and expectations, behavioral patterns and competencies, and environmental influences (see Donovan and Marlatt, 1988, for suggestions), but few of these have been validated with dually diagnosed clients. Modifying, developing, and validating standardized instruments specifically for dually diagnosed clients remains a challenge for researchers. In the meantime, we nonetheless recommend that clinicians use the standardized instruments that do exist such as the Situational Confidence Questionnaire (Annis & Graham, 1988).

Target Areas for Intervention

A detailed assessment of the relevant systems will produce a series of clinical targets for intervention. Here again the process should be collaborative and should stress empirical hypothesis testing of the relationship of substance use to a specific clinical problem. For example, the physiological inquiry may indicate that the dependence syndrome is not a problem, but that substance use is associated with medication noncompliance and that exacerbations of psychosis result. In this case, medication compliance is identified as a target. Similarly, the cognitive investigation may indicate little awareness of the delayed responses to alcohol use. In this case, increasing the client's awareness becomes a target. If the assessment reveals that social anxiety and a lack of social skills are problems, overcoming these difficulties becomes a target. A thorough investigation of all relevant domains will develop numerous specific targets for further elaboration and treatment.

TREATMENT PLANNING

As indicated in Figure 4.1, treatment planning occurs on a different dimension from detection, classification, and specialized assessment.

Treatment planning includes sharing the assessment results with the client, motivating the client for treatment, selecting interventions and goals, and developing a commitment to specific action. The planning process is continuous, dynamic, and longitudinal, one in which client and clinicians, as well as significant others, collaborate over time (Kofoed, 1991). The plan evolves steadily in prescriptiveness as hypotheses are developed, investigated, and translated into specific interventions. The specifics of treatment planning process and treatment for various subgroups of dually diagnosed persons are discussed in Section II. Assessment is ongoing and interactive with treatment planning and treatment.

CONCLUSION

The model of assessment described here depends upon reciprocal feedback loops among the four phases of detection, classification, specialized assessment, and treatment planning. The process is open-ended, dynamic, and continuous with treatment itself; assessment incorporates a series of clinical hypotheses that the team of client, clinicians, and significant others develop, test, and revise over time. The entire assessment assumes that biopsychosocial processes combine and interact in a complex manner to sustain the substance-related behaviors. Assessment addresses all of these elements because successful treatment often involves multiple interventions in different domains.

REFERENCES

Alterman, A.I., Erdlen, D.L., LaPorte, D.J., & Erdlen, F.R. (1982). Effects of illicit drug use in an inpatient psychiatric population. *Addictive Behaviors, 7*, 231–242.

Alterman, A.I., Erdlen, F.R., McLellan, A.T., & Mann, S.C. (1980). Problem drinking in hospitalized schizophrenic patients. *Addictive Behaviors. 5*, 273–276.

Ananth, J., Vandewater, S., Kamal, M., Broksky, A., Gamal, R., & Miller, M. (1989). Missed diagnosis of substance abuse in psychiatric patients. *Hospital and Community Psychiatry. 4*, 297–299.

Annis, H.M., & Graham, J.M. (1988). *Situational Confidence Questionnaire (SCQ-39: Users' Guide*. Toronto: Addiction Research Foundation.

Babor, T.F., Kranzler, H.R., & Lauerman, R.J. (1989). Early detection of harmful alcohol consumption: Comparison of clincal, laboratory, and self-report screening procedures. *Addictive Behaviors. 14*, 139–157.

Babor, T.F., Stephen, R.S., & Marlatt, G.A. (1987). Verbal report methods in clinical research on alcoholism: Reponse bias and its minimization. *Journal of Studies on Alcohol. 48*, 410–424.

Barbee, J.G., Clark, P.D., Crapanzano, M.S., Heintz, G.C., & Kehoe, C.E. (1989). Alcohol and substance abuse among schizophrenic patients presenting to an emergency psychiatric service. *Journal Nervous and Mental Disease. 177*, 400–407.

Blumberg, A.G., Cohen, M., Heaton, A.M., & Klein, D.F. (1971). Covert drug abuse among voluntary hospitalized psychiatric patients. *Journal of the American Medical Association. 217*, 1659–1661.

Dixon, L., Dibietz, E., Myers, P., Conley, R., Medoff, D., & Lehman, A.F. (1993). Comparison of DSM-III-R diagnosis and a brief interview for substance use in state hospital patients. *Hospital and Community Psychiatry. 44*, 748–752.

Dixon, L., Haas, G., Weiden, P., Sweeney, J., & Frances, A. (1990). Acute effects of drug abuse in schizophrenic patients: Clinical observations and patients' self-reports. *Schizophrenia Bulletin. 16*, 69–79.

Donovan, D.M. (1988). Assessment of addictive behaviors: Implications of an emerging biopsychosocial model. In D.M. Donovan & G.M. Marlatt (Eds.), *Assessment of Addictive Behaviors*. (pp. 3–48). New York: Guilford Press.

Donovan, D.M., Kivlahan, D.R., Walker, R.D., & Umlauf, R. (1985). Derivation and validation of neuropsychological clusters among male alcoholics. *Journal of Studies on Alcohol. 46*, 205–211.

Donovan, D.M., & Marlatt, G.A. (Eds.) (1988). *Assessment of Addictive Behavior*. New York: Guilford Press.

Drake, R.E., Alterman, A.I., & Rosenberg, S.R. (1993-a). Detection of substance abuse in persons with severe mental disorders. *Community Mental Health Journal. 29*, 175–192.

Drake, R.E., Bartels, S.J., Teague, G.B., Noordsy, D.L., & Clark, R.E. (1993-b). Treatment of substance abuse in severely mental ill patients. *Journal of Nervous and Mental Disease. 181*, 606–611.

Drake, R.E., Osher, F.C., Noordsy, D.L., Hurlbut, S.C., Teague, G.B., & Beaudett, M.S. (1990). Diagnosis of alcohol use disorders in schizophrenia. *Schizophrenia Bulletin. 16*, 57–67.

Drake, R.E., Osher, F.C., & Wallach, M.A. (1989). Alcohol use and abuse in schizophrenia: A prospective community study. *Journal Nervous and Mental Disease. 177*, 408–414.

Drake, R.E., & Wallach, M.A. (1989). Substance abuse among the chronic mentally ill. *Hospital and Community Psychiatry. 40*, 1041–1046.

Drake, R.E., & Wallach, M.A. (1994). Is moderate drinking realistic for persons with severe mental disorder? *Hospital and Community Psychiatry. 44*, 780–782.

Drake, R.E., Wallach, M.A., Teague, G.B., Freeman, D.H., Paskus, T.S., & Clark, T.A. (1991-a). Housing instability and homelessness among rural schizophrenics. *American Journal of Psychiatry. 148*, 330–336.

Gold, M.S., & Dackis, C.A. (1986). Role of the laboratory in evaluation of suspected drug abusers. *Journal of Clinical Psychiatry. 47*, 17–23.

Kofoed, L.L. (1991). Assessment of comorbid substance abuse and other major psychiatric illnesses. In K. Minkoff & R.E. Drake (Eds.), *Dual Diagnosis of Major Mental Illness and Substance Disorder.* (pp. 43–55). San Francisco: Jossey-Bass.

Kofoed, L.L., & Keys, A. (1988). Using group therapy to persuade dual-diagnosis patients to seek substance abuse treatment. *Hospital and Community Psychiatry. 39*, 1209–1211.

Lehman, A.F., Myers, P., & Corty, E. (1989). Assessment and classification of patients with psychiatric and substance abuse syndromes. *Hospital and Community Psychiatry. 40*, 1019–1025.

Lehman, A.F., Myers, P., Corty, E., & Thompson, J.W. (1994). Prevalence and patterns of 'dual diagnosis' among psychiatric inpatients. *Comprehensive Psychiatry. 35*, 1–5.

Lieberman, J.A., Kinon, B.J., & Loebel, A.D. (1990). Dopaminergic mechanisms in idiopathic and drug-induced psychoses. *Schizophrenia Bulletin. 16*, 97–110.

Lindesmith, A.R. (1968). *Addiction and Opiates.* Chicago: Aldine.

McHugo, G.J., Paskus, T.S., & Drake, R.E. (1993). Detection of alcoholism in schizophrenia using the MAST. *Alcoholism: Clinical and Experimental Research. 17*, 187–191.

Mueser, K.T., Yarnold, P.R., Levinson, D.F., Singh, H., Bellack, A.S., Kee, K., Morrison, R.L., & Yadalam, K.G. (1990). Prevalence of substance abuse in schizophrenia: Demographic and clincial correlates. *Schizophrenia Bulletin. 16*, 31–56.

Osher, F.C., & Kofoed, L.L. (1989). Treatment of patients with both psychiatric and psychoactive substance use disorders. *Hospital and Community Psychiatry. 40*, 1025–1030.

Prochaska, J.O., DiClemente, C.C., & Norcross, J.C. (1992). In search of how people change: Applications to addictive behaviors. *American Psychologist. 47,* 1102–1114.

Regier, D.A., Farmer, M.E., Rae, D.S., Locke, B.Z., Keith, S.J., Judd, L.L., & Goodwin, F.K. (1990). Comorbidity of mental disorders with alcohol and other drug abuse: Results from the Epidemiologic Catchment Area (ECA) Study. *Journal of the American Medical Association. 21,* 2511–2518.

Ries, R.K., & Samson, H. (1987). Substance abuse among inpatient psychiatric patients: Clinical and training issues. *Substance Abuse. 8,* 28–34.

Rosenthal, R.N., Hellerstein, D.J., & Miner, C.R. (1992). Integrated services for treatment of schizophrenic substance abusers: Demographics, symptoms, and substance abuse patterns. *Psychiatric Quarterly. 63,* 3–26.

Safer, D.J. (1987). Substance abuse by young adult chronic patients. *Hospital and Community Psychiatry. 38,* 511–514.

Sevy, S., Kay, S.R., Opler, L.A., & Van Praag, H.M. (1990). Significance of cocaine history in schizophrenia. *Journal of Nervous and Mental Disease. 178,* 642–648.

Skinner, H.A. (1981). Assessment of alcohol problems: Basic principles, critical issues, and future trends. In Y. Israel, F.B. Glaser, H. Kalant, R.E. Popham, W. Schmidt, & R.G. Smart (Eds.), *Research Advances in Alcohol and Drug Problems.* (pp. 319–369).

Stone, A., Greenstein, R., Gamble, G., & McLellan, A.T. (1993). Cocaine use in chronic schizophrenic outpatients receiving depot neuroleptic medications. *Hospital and Community Psychiatry. 44,* 176–177.

Test, M.A., Wallish, L.S., Allness, D.J., & Ripp, K. (1989). Substance use in young adults with schizophrenic disorders. *Schizophrenia Bulletin. 15,* 465–476.

Weiss, R.D., Mirin, S.M., & Griffin, M.L. (1992). Methodological considerations in the diagnosis of coexisting psychiatric disorders in substance abusers. *British Journal of Addiction. 87,* 179–187.

Zinberg, N.E. (1984). *Drug, Set, Setting: The Basis for Controlled Intoxicant Use.* New Haven, CT: Yale University Press.

Section II:

Treatment

5

Overview of Treatment Principles

ROBERT SCHWARTZ and ANTHONY F. LEHMAN

Treatment for persons with comorbid chronic mental illness and substance use disorders must combine and tailor the modalities that are successfully used when these disorders occur separately. Hence, clinicians treating dually diagnosed persons must be conversant with both arrays of treatment modalities. This presents a great challenge. Until recently most clinicians have been trained in the treatment of one disorder to the general exclusion of the other. This chapter offers an overview of the treatment of chronic mental illness and addiction when they appear separately, in order to provide a background to the reader who may be unfamiliar with treatment strategies for one of these types of disorders. Subsequent chapters in this section describe the integrated assessment and treatment of specific subgroups of patients with chronic mental illness and substance abuse.

TREATMENT FOR CHRONIC MENTAL ILLNESS

Chronic mental disorders exert a broad range of effects on the lives of persons whom they afflict. These effects begin with the clinical signs and symptoms currently used to define major mental disorders, including hallucinations, delusions, and disorganized thought processes in schizophrenia and chronic disturbances in mood in manic depressive and major depressive illnesses. However, the effects of these symptoms and underlying impairments in cognitive functioning exert much broader and disabling impacts on these persons' ability to live full and productive lives. Many persons with chronic mental illnesses suffer with impaired interpersonal relationships, reduced role functioning, vocational incapacity, and a lower quality of life.

There now exists considerable consensus which views chronic mental disorders from a vulnerability-stress or biopsychosocial perspective (Zubin & Spring, 1977). This view emphasizes the underlying biological vulnerabilities that predispose an individual to the development of a mental disorder and the importance of psychological and social factors in the onset and course of the disorder. These integrative models form the basis for comprehensive treatment of persons with mental disorders and have set the stage for many exciting therapeutic advances in the treatment of these patients. As a result of their disabilities, these patients have a broad and often daunting range of service needs, which are listed in Table 5.1.

Clinical Psychiatric Treatments: Typical clinical treatment for persons with chronic mental illnesses combines pharmacotherapy with psychological counseling. Pharmacotherapies that significantly reduce symptoms are available for all of the major mental disorders of concern in this volume and form the backbone of treatment for these disorders. As a general rule of thumb, about two-thirds of patients with a mental disorder will have a favorable initial symptom response to appropriate medication. The symptom response rates in the literature for antipsychotic medications, antidepressants, and anti-manics (e.g., lithium) are all in the 65–70% range (Kaplan & Sadock, 1985).

In recent years pharmacotherapeutic strategies have been developed for patients who do not respond to these conventional medications. For schizophrenia, new classes of antipsychotics are

Table 5.1. Range of Service Needs
for Persons with
Severe Mental Illness

Clinical psychiatric treatment
Family services
Rehabilitation services
Housing services
Income supports
Legal services
General medical care
Dental care

being developed and are proving useful for treating patients who do not respond to the conventional antipsychotics, such as haloperidol (Haldol), fluphenazine (Prolixin), chlorpromazine (Thorazine), and thiothixene (Navane). Examples of these novel antipsychotics include clozapine (Clozaril), and risperidone (Risperdal). Approximately 30% of patients who do not respond to the conventional antipsychotics respond favorably to clozapine (Kane, et al., 1988). Similarly, new classes of antidepressants have been developed which offer additional options when the older classes of antidepressants, the tricyclics and the monoamine oxidase inhibitors, fail or have adverse side effects. These newer antidepressants, selective serotonin reuptake inhibitors, include fluoxitene (Prozac), sertraline (Zoloft) and paroxetine (Paxil). Finally, for those patients with manic-depressive illness who do not respond to or suffer unacceptable side effects from lithium, the anticonvulsants, valproic acid (Depakote) and carbamazepine (Tegretol), are often effective.

Symptom reduction is a major, but not the only goal of clinical treatment for chronic mental disorders. These illnesses have devastating effects on an individual's self-esteem and morale, which may in part account for the high suicide rates among these patients, as high as 10% (Kaplan & Sadock, 1985). Furthermore this demoralization contributes to poor compliance with treatment, thus creating a downward cycle. The main goal of psychological interventions for patients with these disorders is to reduce demoralization, enhance the patient's capacity to cope with the illness and improve self-esteem.

Psychological treatments for chronic mental illnesses include both individual and group therapies. Current practice emphasizes a supportive mode of counseling, which encompasses empathic listening, active problem solving around issues of everyday life, education about the illness and treatment, and a generally supportive relationship with the therapist (Wasylenki, 1992). This can be provided either individually or in groups. The theory underlying this approach is that mental illness impairs the patient's capacity to relate to others and to recognize and cope with stresses that may result in relapse or other problems. The purpose of the therapeutic relationship is to offset these deficits with emotional support, practical advice and training about everyday life, and enduring contact with someone who is objective, yet knows and cares about the patient.

Certain potential benefits of supportive therapy can be identified. The supportive therapeutic relationship provides a context to educate the patient about the illness, the role of prescribed medications, and the importance of recognizing early signs of relapse. The net effect is a more individualized approach to pharmacotherapy, which in turn may yield better medication compliance and symptom control.

Support and practical advice can also help to reduce the distress experienced by these patients in the course of everyday life problems. Failure to deal effectively with such stresses can lead to symptom relapse. Thoughtful listening and suggestions from the therapist can enhance the patient's sense of hope and competence in the face of these problems. Patient education about the association of symptoms with stress and the importance of managing distress can improve the patient's sense of control and ability to cope.

A more specific and structured type of group treatment that has developed in recent years is *social skills training* (Anthony & Liberman, 1986). Largely designed by investigators at the UCLA Center for Schizophrenia and Psychiatric Rehabilitation, these social skill training groups target the social disabilities that accompany chronic mental illness. This technique utilizes structured behavioral techniques, including role-playing, modeling, feedback, rehearsal, behavioral coaching and rewards to enhance patients' skill levels. The types of skills taught vary widely and include communication skills (listening, processing, and sending), assertiveness skills, problem-solving skills, and skills related to specific activities of daily living (medication management, shopping, use of transportation, money management, leisure time activities, and use of community resources).

Family Interventions

During the past decade a variety of family interventions have been described based upon the premise that families of persons with chronic mental illnesses need support, information, practical advice, and training in how to cope with the challenges posed by these illnesses. Several types of family interventions have been developed to help families cope with chronic mental illness (McFarlane, 1983; Anderson, Reiss & Hogarty, 1986). These programs differ in terms of various characteristics, but share a common focus on educating the family about chronic mental illness and treatment and assisting the family in the resolution of everyday problems that arise because of the illness.

Rehabilitation

With the mass relocation over the past four decades of the locus of care for persons with chronic mental illnesses from the hospital to the community, there has been an explosive growth of community-based psychosocial rehabilitation and support programs for these patients. These include: a) vocational rehabilitation services; and b) psychosocial rehabilitation centers.

Programs to improve the work functioning of these persons have existed for a long time, dating back to the rural public asylums of the last century, which often included a farm on which patients worked. In more recent times this concern about work has translated into various types of vocational rehabilitation programs. The types of programs include hospital-based workshop programs, lodge programs with a focus on work, sheltered workshops, vocational counseling programs, job clubs, psychosocial clubhouse programs, and supportive employment. These programs can be subsumed under two general types: *"train and place"* programs and *"place and train"* programs.

The traditional "train and place" model, which includes all transitional and sheltered vocational rehabilitation programs, first assesses and trains the patient with regard to general work habits and particular job skills. The patients are assessed for their work aptitudes and preferences, assisted in improving their work habits, and *trained* to do a certain kind of work. Once they have achieved a certain level of competence and consistent performance, they are *"placed"* at a regular job site. The advantages of this model are that it provides the opportunity to assess and work with the patients before they are exposed to the rigors of a real job setting and takes advantage of the efficiency of serving large numbers of patients in a rehabilitation center. The major problems with this model are that it may not adequately prepare patients for the transition from the shelter of the rehabilitation center to the regular work world, patient choices about the types of work are limited, and the duration of training delays the time until they can begin to earn a wage.

In response to these problems a new model of vocational rehabilitation has developed in recent years, the *"place and train"* model. Under this approach, patients work with a vocational counselor to identify their vocational goals and the type of job they would like to have which fits with their abilities. Patients are then *placed* at an actual job site and are *trained* to do that specific job in that specific setting. Under this model, often referred to as "supported employment," the patient works with a job coach who assists the patient in whatever way is necessary to learn and keep that job. The advantages of this approach are that it is highly individualized, avoids the stressful transition from sheltered to unsheltered work settings, and allows patients to begin earning a wage more quickly. The disadvantages are its costs and the dependence upon employers who are willing to support this type of on-the-job training for disabled persons.

At least four organized models of psychosocial rehabilitation can be identified: the Fountain House Clubhouse Model, the Fairweather Lodge, the Boston University Model, and the UCLA Social Skills Training Model (Anthony & Liberman, 1986). Fountain House, founded in 1948 in New York City, is one of oldest and best known psychosocial rehabilitation programs in the United States. This model seeks to enhance patients' sense of hope and competence through self-help, assisted by staff and other supports as needed. The Fairweather Lodge model began during the 1960's as a response to the problem of recidivism among patients discharged from the hospital. Small groups of patients in the hospital are formed and taught daily living, coping, and work skills. They are encouraged to function as semi-autonomous groups, fostering mutual responsibility and learning the skills necessary to live in the community. When ready the group moves *together* into a community lodge with a home-like setting where they function essentially as a family.

Two major centers for the development of psychosocial rehabilitation methods for chronic mental illness are the Boston University Center for Psychiatric Rehabilitation and the UCLA Center for Chronic Mental Illness and Psychiatric Rehabilitation. These programs emphasize behavioral and social learning theories to develop specific packages and programs to teach patients social and community living skills.

Housing and Other Services

Housing services are perhaps one of the most important yet least studied aspect of psychosocial interventions for persons with chronic mental illness. Considerable variety characterizes the continuum of community residential care settings for persons with chronic mental illness, and the literature is replete with various terminologies for referring to these settings. One general paradigm is the "linear continuum" of housing under which patients move through a series of increasingly independent settings. This continuum includes transitional halfway houses, long-term group residences, cooperative apartments, intensive care community residences, and board and care homes.

Due to a variety of problems with this "linear" continuum paradigm, a second major shift in housing for persons with chronic mental illness is now underway. This is referred to as the "paradigm of supported housing" (Ridgway & Zipple, 1990). This paradigm emphasizes mainstream housing settings integrated fully into the community with support services provided as needed, but not on-site. Housing is conceived as a normal living environment, not a treatment or service setting. Because this paradigm emphasizes individual choice and normalization of the patient's living environment, it has attracted considerable attention and advocacy throughout the country.

Because of the disabling effects of mental illness, these persons often require income support. The major Federal programs for this are Social Security Disability Insurance (SSDI), which is for persons who were gainfully employed at some time but became disabled, and Supplemental Security Income (SSI) for persons who have never had significant gainful employment because of disability. Patients with cognitive impairments typically need assistance in successfully completing the application processes for these entitlements.

Consumer Self-Help

A major change occurring in service for persons with chronic mental illnesses is the growth of self-help programs. One of the great misconceptions about persons with chronic mental illnesses is that they are unable to help themselves, and too often they are treated as incompetent to make decisions. In response to this stigma, a significant self-help and consumer advocacy movement has grown in this country in recent years. In addition to public advocacy, this movement has spawned a variety of self-help programs and activities for persons with chronic mental illnesses. These include informal social clubs and drop-in centers, which primarily provide a place to go, social contact, and natural support. More recently there has been a considerable growth in direct involvement of "consumers" in the provision of services (Van Tosh, 1993). Such programs employ consumers as direct service providers, such as in community survival skills training and advocacy, as well as bridging agents between the patient and service professionals. While the best ways to integrate consumers into direct service provision are still being worked out, when done well this involvement adds tremendously to the capacity of service programs to engage patients and to tailor services to individual needs.

Integrating Services

The complex array of services needed by persons with mental illnesses has led to considerable attention on how best to integrate these services. "Case management" now commands wide conceptual acceptance as a bulwark for organizing effective services for persons with chronic mental illness.

A wide variety of potential activities have been subsumed under the term, case management. These include outreach, patient assessment, case planning, referral to service providers, advocacy for the patient, direct casework, developing natural support systems, reassessment, advocacy for resource development, monitoring quality, public education, and crisis intervention. Case management can be provided by individuals, teams, or systems. The great variability in the definition of the dimensions of case management contributes to much of the ambiguity and confusion that exists in the field.

The best known example of an intensive model of clinical case management is assertive community treatment developed in Madison, Wisconsin (Stein & Test, 1980). In a fourteen month randomized comparison of hospital treatment plus standard aftercare versus an innovative, assertive, outreach and community based treatment program, the patients in the experimental program had lower rates of hospitalization, higher levels of functioning, greater life satisfaction and no differences in levels of family burden compared to the control cases. Costs for the two programs were essentially equivalent. These results have been replicated elsewhere. Other studies of case management models have produced similar results (Olfson, 1990).

Together these studies indicate that under the right circumstances with appropriately targeted patients, intensive case management can be highly effective in sustaining patients with mental illness in the community and enhancing outcomes. However, case management is not a panacea. The major unanswered questions pertain to which patients require this type of service at what intensity and at what time points during their illness.

Locus of Care

In this era of brief hospitalization, psychosocial treatments occur primarily in community-based settings, including clinics, private offices, day treatment programs, psychosocial rehabilitation centers, vocational rehabilitation centers, and residential care settings. Indeed research on alternatives to long-term hospitalization for persons with chronic mental illness has shown no advantages to extended hospital care when community-based care is a feasible alternative (Braun, 1981). Even in the community, however, new pressures are arising to shift the locus of care further from centers of treatment to mainstream community contexts, such as mobile treatment teams, home-based family counseling, "place-and train" vocational services, and supported housing.

TREATMENT FOR SUBSTANCE USE DISORDERS

Psychoactive substance use, abuse and dependence (addiction) exist along a continuum of severity. Cautious social use of alcohol is common in our society, and generally not considered problematic. Use of other psychoactive substances (excluding nicotine and caffeine) is illegal, and hence problematic. Whether use begins with a legal or an illegal substance, some users develop substance related problems over time, which may lead to a diagnosis of a psychoactive substance use disorder, either abuse or dependence.

A clinical model useful in thinking about addiction is that it, like mental illness, is a biopsychosocial illness. Addiction is a chronic, progressive, relapsing illness which can be fatal if untreated. It deleteriously affects many aspects of a patient's life. The craving and compulsive use in spite of adverse consequences can lead to serious problems in a patient's physical or mental health, legal status, relationships, occupation, finances and spiritual life. Fortunately, addiction can be treated successfully. Treatment consists of various modalities which are provided across a spectrum of settings. These settings vary in their restrictiveness, intensity and cost, and are matched to the stage and acuity of the illness.

Treatment Settings

a) *Inpatient and Residential Care*: Addicted persons require inpatient detoxification when they are unable to stop using drugs on an outpatient basis, or if their medical or psychiatric condition make an outpatient attempt at abstinence dangerous. Untreated alcohol or sedative hypnotic withdrawal (e.g. alprazolam (Xanax), diazepam (Valium)) can lead to seizures, delirium and even death. While opiate withdrawal in itself is not life threatening, unremitting opiate addiction can lead to death from overdose or medical complications. Therefore, opiate inpatient detoxification can also be life saving if it motivates the patient towards abstinence. Treatment in a detoxification unit may include medication to safely manage withdrawal, medical assessment, substance abuse education, and an aftercare referral.

After detoxification, patients may attend an inpatient rehabilitation program. These generally consist of a structured program based on 12-step recovery programs (Alcoholics Anonymous, 1976). They offer group therapy, individual counseling, education, relapse prevention techniques, and Alcoholic Anonymous (AA) and Narcotics Anonymous (NA) meeting. They may also have adjunctive behavioral, spiritual, medical and psychological therapies. These programs were initially designed to last 28 days. However, due to cost constraints, their length of stay now is often shorter.

Halfway houses for persons with an addiction are time-limited, and targeted for those who are not ready to return to their previous living arrangement or who lack housing which would support their sobriety. They may be accessed after an inpatient rehabilitation program. Residents are encouraged to obtain employment and participate in a 12-step recovery program (Geller, 1992).

Residential and inpatient programs offer the advantage of removing the person temporarily from an environment that supports substance use.

b) *Outpatient:* Day hospitals offer milieu, group and individual treatments similar to rehabilitation programs. The patients, however, return home or to supportive housing in the evening. They are time-limited and serve as an alternative to inpatient care and a bridge to less intense outpatient services.

Comprehensive outpatient services offer methadone and "drug free" treatment, although these modalities are often found as separate programs. These programs generally include a combination of individual, group or family therapy, and medication (e.g. antabuse, methadone or anti-depressants). Persons with an addiction are usually also referred to self-help groups. Urine drug screening and breathalyzer testing for alcohol use are essential ingredients in any outpatient substance abuse treatment. They provide an objective measure of use. This is necessary because the guilt, shame, denial or potential adverse legal or occupational consequences of relapse may be obstacles to early help-seeking. It also is helpful to document a patient's recovery for employment or legal purposes.

Treatment Modalities

A variety of treatment modalities are employed across inpatient, residential, and outpatient settings. These include: individual, group or family therapy, medication and self help.

a) *Individual Therapy*: There is little empirical information to assist the clinician in deciding which persons with addiction will benefit from individual therapy, or when in the natural history of the illness it is indicated (Rounsaville & Carroll, 1992). Nevertheless, clinical practice indicates it can be useful to either motivate the patient for treatment, work on specific issues that may be difficult to deal with initially in group, or as an adjunct to other modalities.

During active substance use and early recovery, the goals of individual therapy are to teach patients about the disease of addiction, help them shift their identity to that of an addict (Brown, 1985), and to stop using psychoactive substances. Controlled drug use is often the patient's fantasy. Early in the course of treatment it may be necessary for the patient to have several unsuccessful attempts at controlled use to accept its futility.

Discovering patients' explanations for loss of control over substances can be useful. Persons with addiction may believe if the "problem causing their addiction" could be treated, they would no longer be addicted, and could return to "social use." Patients' explanations for loss of control frequently include having an underlying emotional disturbance, family problems, too much stress, not enough willpower, the wrong job, and a myriad of others. Knowing patients' own conceptual model of their problem helps the therapist direct and educate them in an attempt to accept the biopsychosocial illness model as at least partially responsible for their addiction (Brower, Blow, & Beresford, 1989). If this is successful, patients will find it easier to accept responsibility for their treatment.

In early recovery, relapse prevention techniques play an essential role. The AA slogan "keep away from people, places and things" related to addiction is a simple eloquent example. Brown (1985) recommends emphasizing positive actions to replace the addictive behaviors. These may include calling an AA sponsor, going to AA or group therapy meetings, and reading recovery literature (Alcoholics Anonymous, 1976).

Marlatt and Gordon (1985) recommend cognitive/behavioral interventions to identify and deal with relapse triggers. These triggers can include peer pressure, exposure to the drug or paraphernalia, and painful affects (Daly, Moss & Campbell, 1987). Relapse is frequently part of the natural history of the addiction. Therefore Marlatt suggests having a relapse plan ready, which can be put into effect if necessary. This would prevent a "slip," without adverse consequences, from becoming a full blown relapse. Gorski (1989) also has been a pioneer in practical relapse prevention techniques.

While there are many roads to recovery from addiction, many patients find 12-step meetings essential. Discussion of the patient's participation in AA/NA is an important part of therapy. The therapist must become familiar with AA/NA literature, slogans and meetings. Patients' use of AA must be explored. How often are they attending, what types of meetings, do they have a home group and a sponsor? These should be part of the basic evaluation, and ongoing inquiry. Resistance to AA attendance or obtaining a sponsor should be explored and clarified.

b) *Group Therapy*: This modality is particularly useful to reduce social isolation, denial, manipulation, projection, and overdependence on the therapist early in individual therapy. Education groups are generally offered at the onset of treatment. They allow the patient time to acclimate to a group setting without much initial demand for interaction. It also supplies the patient with essential information about the disease and recovery process.

Group therapy in early recovery is generally task-oriented with a focus on here-and-now issues related directly to addiction. Topics may include identification of feeling states as a relapse trigger, euphoric recall (where persons with addictions only remember the "high" of their active drug use), interpersonal behavior, and practical problems dealing with a sober life.

c) *Family Therapy*: The major schools of systemic family therapy can be adapted for substance abuse treatment. Multiple family techniques have been utilized with this population as well (Kaufman, 1991).

Intervention techniques (Johnson, 1980) are used to motivate persons with addiction into treatment. The clinician gathers key members (e.g. family, employer, friends, physician) of the patient's social network. Rehearsing a group confrontation without the patient, they each in turn review specific problematic events caused by alcohol or drugs. During the actual intervention, the message is one of caring, coupled with a wish for the patient to get help. Treatment (often inpatient) is arranged prior to the intervention, so it can be immediately accessed.

"Co-dependency" (Beattie, 1987) occurs when the behavior of a person is controlled by the other person's addiction. The co-dependent person feels responsible for the addicted person's behavior and drinking. Persons with co-dependency enable addiction to progress by protecting addicted persons from the consequences of their behavior. It is often difficult for family members or treatment staff not to "help" the persons with an addiction out of their predicaments. Yet, it may be precisely these negative consequences that drive the patient towards the decision to quit. Successful treatment usually requires dealing with this issue. Al-Anon, a 12-step support group, is often a useful resource for the families of persons with addiction.

"Enabling" refers to the more general phenomenon of actions by others that inadvertently reinforce the patient's addictive behaviors. Usually the motivation for the enabling behavior is to protect or help the patient. Examples of enabling include calling the addicted person's employer to make excuses for absence due to addiction or giving addicted persons money for food because they spent all of their money on drugs. These actions, while well intended, allow addicted persons to avoid the consequences of their behaviors and hence enable them to continue to deny problems and to use substances.

d) *Medications*: Medications for addiction have been less well developed than for chronic mental disorders. The benzodiazepines are a safe and effective means for detoxifying patients dependent on alcohol. Methadone, a synthetic narcotic agonist, and the anti-hypertensive clonidine (Catapress) are both safe and effective means of detoxifying patients from opiates.

Methadone maintenance has proven itself in numerous studies to be an extremely effective outpatient treatment (Cooper, 1981) for heroin addiction. It relieves drug craving, and at adequate doses, blocks heroin's euphoric effect. Methadone is administered orally in specially licensed clinics, which must provide counseling, and medical evaluation. Adjunctive services such as family therapy, vocational, educational assessment and referral may be offered as well. Opiate antagonists such as naltrexone (Trexan) have not been used widely. They have a high dropout rate, and may be better suited to highly motivated individuals.

The pharmacologic treatment of cocaine dependence has not yet lived up to its promise. A variety of medications including carbamazepine, desipramine, fluoxetine, and bromocriptine have been studied. However, many of the studies have been preliminary (Meyer, 1992). Despite the passage of ten years since the first forays into pharmacologic treatment of cocaine dependence, these treatments remain investigational.

Antabuse (disulfiram) interferes with aldehyde dehydrogenase, leading to build up of acetaldehyde when alcohol is consumed. This results in nausea, vomiting, flushing, headache, tachycardia, and hypotension which can lead to shock and death. Knowing the serious side effects may deter some patients taking Antabuse from impulsive drinking. However, if they have decided to drink again, they can drink after discontinuing the medication for several days. Antabuse is most effective in highly motivated individuals, or when ingested under observation, such as by a family member.

e) *Self-Help*: Narcotics Anonymous, Cocaine Anonymous and other 12-step self-help groups are based on the principles of Alcoholics Anonymous. Founded by two chronic alcoholics, Bill W. and Dr. Bob in 1935, it since grown to a large international membership numbering over 170,000.

The only requirement to be a member of AA is to wish to stop drinking. It is a self-supporting organization that has no political or religious affiliations. The AA Program consists of learning and applying the twelve steps (Table 5.2) through various types of meetings and literature. A powerful 24 hour/day support network is available to members. New members are encouraged to ask for a sponsor at a meeting. These are sober members who have worked the program for some time and can serve as a guide.

Spirituality, represented in part by the concept of a higher power, is an important part of the program. A higher power is a force, other than oneself, that helps the persons with addiction in the struggle over the loss of control. This higher power, chosen by the individual, may or may not be God.

CONCLUSION

The nature of addiction and severe mental illness as well as their treatments share many commonalities as well as important differences. Both addiction and chronic mental illness can be usefully viewed as biopsychosocial disorders in which biological, psychological, and social factors influence both the onset and course of the disorders. Both are persistent problems with which persons must cope in some way for most of their lives and which lead to quite variable levels of disability and recovery.

Table 5.2. Twelve Steps of Alcoholics Anonymous

---

1. We admitted we were powerless over alcohol — that our lives had become unmanageable.
2. Came to believe that a Power greater than ourselves could restore us to sanity.
3. Made a decision to turn our will and our lives over to the care of God as we understood him.
4. Made a searching and fearless moral inventory of ourselves.
5. Admitted to God, to ourselves, and to another human being the exact nature of our wrong doings.
6. Were entirely ready to have God remove all these defects of character.
7. Humbly asked him to remove our shortcomings.
8. Made a list of all persons we had harmed, and became willing to make amends to them all.
9. Made direct amends to such people wherever possible, except when to do so would injure them or others.
10. Continued to take personal inventory and when we were wrong promptly admitted it.
11. Sought through prayer and meditation to improve our conscious contact with God as we understood him, praying only for knowledge of His will for us and the power to carry that out.
12. Having had a spiritual awakening as the result of these steps, we tried to carry this message to alcoholics, and to practice these principals in all our affairs.

Source: *Twelve Steps and Twelve Traditions*. New York, AA World Services, Inc, New York, 1978.

Because both types of disorders are persistent and are typically met initially by patients and families with denial and shame, early phases of treatment must emphasize engagement of patients and their families in the therapeutic process and education about the illness and possible treatments. Treatment options for both types of disorders typically include a combination of medical intervention, psychological counseling, family support, and environmental support and intervention (housing, financial, legal services, for example). Treatment must be viewed as ongoing over many years, varying in intensity depending upon course, and with the realistic expectation that relapses are to be expected. The philosophy of "one day at a time" applies to the recovery process from both addiction and chronic mental illness.

The primary difference between the treatments for these disorders relate to prevailing philosophies. The biopsychosocial illness model is more accepted for mental illness than for addiction, which still tends to be viewed as much as a moral as a medical problem by society. The efficacy of medications for mental illness is better established than for addiction, and therefore one will encounter more controversy in addiction treatment settings about the use of medications. Psychological treatments for addiction tend to be more confrontational whereas those for chronic mental illness tend to be more supportive.

The practitioner treating persons with dual diagnosis must be prepared to deal with these commonalities and differences because treatment for these persons inevitably requires a team effort. A team that works from a common perspective will be more successful, and therefore time will be well spent to explore areas of shared and divergent views. Given the ambiguities in the field, the goal for a team should be to proceed with open and informed minds, respecting the valid divergence of opinions among team members, and seeking what works best for the individual patient, not allowing ideology to overwhelm good clinical judgment.

REFERENCES

Alcoholics Anonymous. (1976). New York: AA World Services, Inc.

Anderson, C.M., Reiss, D.J., & Hogarty, G.E. (1986). *Chronic Mental Illness and the Family*. New York: Guilford Press.

Anthony, W.A., & Liberman, R.P. (1986). The practice of psychiatric rehabilitation: historical, conceptual, and research base. *Chronic Mental Illness Bulletin. 12*, 542–559.

Beattie, M. (1987). *Co-Dependent No More*. New York: Harper & Row.

Braun, P., Kochansky, G., Shapiro, R., Greenberg, S., Gudeman, J.E., Johnson, S., & Shore, M.F. (1981). Overview: deinstitutionalization of psychiatric patients: a critical review of outcome studies. *American Journal of Psychiatry. 138*, 736–749.

Brower, K.J., Blow, F.C., & Beresford, T.P. (1989). Treatment implications of chemical dependency models: an integrative approach. *Journal of Substance Abuse Treatment. 6*, 147–157.

Brown, S. (1985). *Treating The Alcoholic. A Developmental Model of Recovery*. New York; John Wiley & Sons.

Cooper, J.R. (1989). Methadone treatment and acquired immunodeficiency syndrome. *Journal of the American Medical Association. 262*, 1664–1681.

Daly, D.C., & Moss, H., & Campbell, F. (1987). *Dual Disorders, Counseling Clients with Chemical Dependency and Mental Illness*. Center City, Minn: Hazelden.

Geller, A. (1992). Rehabilitation programs and halfway houses. In J.H. Lowinson, P. Ruiz, R.B. Millman (Eds). *Substance Abuse, A Comprehensive Textbook*. 2nd ed, Baltimore: Williams and Wilkins.

Gorski, T.T. (1989). *Passages Through Recovery*. Center City, Minn: Hazelden.

Johnson, V.E. (1980). *I'll Quit Tommorrow*. San Francisco: Harper & Row.

Kane, J., Honigfeld, G., Singer, J., Meltzer, H.Y., & the Clozaril Collaborative Study Group (1988). Clozapine for the treatment-resistant schizophrenic. *Archives of General Psychiatry. 45*, 789–796.

Kaplan, H.I., & Sadock, B.J. (1985). *Comprehensive Textbook of Psychiatry/IV*. Baltimore: Williams and Wilkins.

Kaufman, E. (1991). The family in drug and alcohol addiction. In N.S. Miller (Ed.). *Comprehensive Handbook of Drug and Alcohol Addiction*. New York: Marcel Dekker Inc.

Marlatt, G.A., & Gordon, J. (Eds.) (1985). *Relapse Prevention*. New York: Guilford Press.

McFarlane, W.R. (Ed.). (1983). *Family Therapy in Chronic mental illness*. New York: Guilford.

Meyer, R.E. (1992). New pharmacotherapies for cocaine dependence ... revisited. *Archives of General Psychiatry. 49*, 900–904.

Olfson, M. (1990). Assertive community treatment: an evaluation of the experimental evidence. *Hospital and Community Psychiatry. 41*, 634–641.

Ridgway, P., & Zipple, A.M. (1990). The paradigm shift in residential services: from the linear continuum to supported housing approaches. *Psychosocial Rehabilitation Journal. 13*, 11–31.

Rounsaville, B.J., & Carrol, K.M. (1992). Individual Psychotherapy for Drug Abusers, In J.H. Lowinson, P. Ruiz & R.B. Millman. *Substance Abuse, A Comprehensive Textbook*. 2nd ed, Baltimore: Williams & Wilkins.

Stein, L., & Test, M.A. (1980). An alternative to mental hospital treatment I: conceptual model, treatment program, and clinical evaluation. *Archives of General Psychiatry*. 37, 392–397.

Van Tosh, L. (1993). *Working for a Change. Employment of Consumers/Servivors in the Design and Provision of Services for Persons Who Are Homeless and Mentally Disabled*. Rockville, MD: Center for Mental Health Services.

Wasylenki, D.A. (1992). Psychotherapy of chronic mental illness revisited. *Hospital Community Psychiatry*. 43, 123–127.

Zubin, J., & Spring, B. (1977). Vulnerability: a new view of chronic mental illness. *Journal of Abnormal Psychology*. 86, 103–126.

6

Treatment of Substance Use Disorders and Schizophrenia

KATE BERGMANN CAREY

This chapter provides a guide to the treatment of substance abuse in persons with schizophrenia. Treatment of persons with both schizophrenia and substance abuse (SSAs) poses many challenges. First, no cure exists for either disorder. Thus, appropriate treatment goals include abstinence from non-prescribed drugs and alcohol, and stability or remission of the psychiatric disorder. Success, however, is usually measured in the degree of approximation to these goals. Second, both schizophrenia and substance abuse can severely impair adaptive function. In combination, these conditions disable individuals in their ability to fulfill important societal roles such as parent, spouse, wage earner, and citizen. Third, a tradition of separate mental health and substance abuse services restricts the ability of existing treatment resources to meet the challenge. Systems components such as staff training, administrative structure, reimbursement policies, and treatment philosophies are organized around treating disorders rather than treating people. Finally, the majority of treatment for these disorders takes place on an outpatient basis. This limits the degree of control exercised by treatment personnel over critical variables affecting treatment, such as availability of substances and compliance with treatment recommendations.

Acknowledging these difficulties, this chapter takes an outpatient treatment planning perspective, with appropriate references to integrating inpatient and outpatient services. Because of these and related challenges, treatment of persons with SSA continues to be an endeavor inspired by creative problem solving in the field, with recent support from clinical research. Guidelines contained in this chapter draw on both sources of knowledge.

PATTERNS OF CO-OCCURRENCE

As discussed in Chapter 2, substance abuse occurs more frequently among persons with schizophrenia than in the general population. The Epidemiological Catchment Area Study indicates that *lifetime* prevalence of substance abuse/dependence diagnoses among persons with schizophrenia is 47%, compared to 16.7% in the general population (Regier et al., 1990). Persons with schizophrenia exceed all other psychiatric diagnostic groups in the percentage of comorbid substance abuse/dependence diagnoses. The prevalence of *recent* abuse in clinical samples ranges from 20% to 40% (Mueser, Bellack, & Blanchard, 1992).

The co-occurrence of schizophrenia and substance abuse is complicated by heterogeneity from at least four sources. First, there is considerable heterogeneity among individuals with schizophrenia (e.g., Heinrichs, 1993). Differences in premorbid functioning, symptom severity, response to pharmacologic treatment, and degree of residual impairment between acute episodes represent just a few of the factors that can affect the course of treatment and prognosis. Second, the pharmacologic effects of abused substances vary considerably. Some stimulate or depress the central nervous system, whereas others have the capacity to mimic psychotic-like states. Clinical surveys indicate that alcohol, cannabis, and stimulants are the substances abused most often by persons with schizophrenia (e.g., Mueser et al., 1990). Even this subset represents varying routes of administration, intoxication and withdrawal symptoms.

Third, persons with SSA vary in their degree of involvement with substances. Treatment providers see persons with schizophrenia whose substance use ranges from occasional and opportunistic, to more classically defined addiction patterns. Finally, a great deal of variability exists in the nature of functional impairment resulting from substance use. Some persons with schizophrenia manifest poor outcomes with minimal substance use (Drake, Osher, & Wallace, 1989), whereas others can use marijuana or alcohol on a daily basis without relapsing. The latter are probably underrepresented in the literature (Dixon, Haas, Weiden, Sweeney, & Frances, 1990); these patients give mixed reports of symptom exacerbation and amelioration as a result of their substance use. In summary, the heterogeneity inherent in the co-occurrence of schizophrenia and substance abuse suggests that treatment approaches must be flexible and tailored to the needs of the individual.

PHARMACOLOGIC TREATMENTS

The pharmacologic treatment for schizophrenia involves use of neuroleptic drugs. These drugs reduce or eliminate positive symptoms of schizophrenia for many clients; they also effectively treat substance-induced psychoses in persons without schizophrenia. Thus, neuroleptics serve as the cornerstone of both acute treatment and maintenance therapy for persons with SSA (see Siris, 1990). However, the use of neuroleptic medications for schizophrenia in the context of active substance abuse raises important concerns, including (a) potentially harmful drug interactions, (b) difficulties in achieving optimal dosages of neuroleptic medication, and (c) the potential of prescribed drugs to be abused.

Many treatment providers express concern about mixing psychiatric medications with a potentially unknown combination of street drugs. This is an important treatment consideration that should be communicated clearly to the client. However, unless a client is known to be abusing a drug with clear risk of negative interaction with his/her neuroleptic regimen, the benefits of controlling schizophrenic symptoms suggest that the appropriate neuroleptic regimen ought to be used.

It can be difficult to determine the optimal dose that balances the benefits and risks of this class of drugs. On the one hand, undermedication is a risk, due to the well-documented problem of medication noncompliance among persons with SSA (e.g., Drake et al., 1989). Many persons with SSA report that they discontinue their medications when they plan to drink in an attempt to avoid drug interactions (Pristach & Smith, 1990). As a result, it is often unclear whether relapses are due to substance use, lack of medication, or a combination of both. Depot administration of neuroleptics can be an effective way of reducing compliance problems for clients with SSA.

On the other hand, overuse of neuroleptics with actively abusing clients is another risk. Active abuse may exacerbate baseline levels of psychotic disorganization, requiring higher doses of medication to control symptoms. In addition to the long-term risk of tardive diskinesia, acute consequences of overmedication include sedation, parkinsonian side effects, akathisia, and akinesia. These uncomfortable side effects of neuroleptic treatment may motivate persons with SSA to use street drugs or alcohol to counteract them. Appropriate medication dosages should be determined in a drug-free state. Toward this end, an extended inpatient stay may be valuable for periodic dose adjustment.

Abuse of prescribed medications represents an additional concern. Many substance abusing clients become amateur pharmacists; just as they tinker with types and dosages of street drugs and alcohol to achieve desired effects, they may do so with their prescribed medications. For example, side effects of neuroleptic medications are often treated with anticholinergic agents. However, anticholinergic medications have abuse potential, producing a pleasant euphoria. Some clients will use up their medications earlier than expected, or lose their prescriptions periodically and request additional medication. Patterns of behavior such as these should be addressed, to determine if the medication is being abused by either the client or his/her associates.

Mood and anxiety disturbances have been independently associated with both schizophrenia and substance abuse. Tricyclic antidepressants and lithium can be used with persons with SSA. However, the erratic treatment attendance characteristic of SSA clients may interfere with adequate monitoring of blood levels of lithium. MAO inhibitors should not be used with clients who are actively abusing substances or at risk for relapse, due to the risk of hypertensive crisis. Benzodiazepines are frequently used to treat adjunctive anxiety. Pharmacological treatment may be justified in cases of extreme anxiety, or for clients who are not able to participate in behavioral anxiety reduction strategies. However, the substantial abuse potential of benzodiazepines requires (a) serious consideration of alternative strategies for anxiety treatment, (b) short-term treatment, and (c) careful monitoring.

Finally, pharmacologic treatments employed to reduce substance use can be considered for use with persons with SSA as one component of a comprehensive treatment package. Methadone may have antipsychotic properties; thus clients who receive methadone as part of their treatment for opiate addiction may require lower doses of neuroleptics. Disulfiram (Antabuse) is used to help alcoholics maintain abstinence. Because disulfiram can exacerbate psychosis it should be used with caution (Ban, 1977). However, it can be considered, especially if the client has used it with success in the past. Banys (1988) suggests beginning with reduced dosages and monitoring levels of thought disorder and disorientation.

In summary, the benefits of treating a psychotic disorder with neuroleptics usually outweigh the risks of interactions with abused substances. However, clients must be educated about these risks, and in the context of active substance abuse, optimal dosages of psychiatric medications should be periodically reevaluated. For clients known to abuse street drugs and/or alcohol, abuse of prescribed drugs (especially anticholinergic and antianxiety agents) is also a risk. Medications designed to reduce substance use directly are most effective as adjuncts to psychosocial treatments.

PSYCHOSOCIAL TREATMENT

Treatment of substance abuse disorders in persons with schizophrenia must include a well-conceived psychosocial component. The approach recommended in this chapter is based on a model advanced by Osher and Kofoed (1989). These authors proposed a model of dual diagnosis treatment containing the following phases: engagement, persuasion, active treatment, and relapse prevention. *Engagement* refers to the process of connecting clients with treatment. *Persuasion* refers to the process of convincing the client that substance abuse is the cause of problems and that abstinence is a desirable goal. *Active treatment* refers to the aspects of treatment explicitly designed to attain and maintain abstinence. Once a client expresses a desire to stop drinking or drugging, he/she must develop the skills, the attitudes, and the support system to achieve that goal. Finally, the *relapse preven-*

tion phase acknowledges the fact that recovery is an ongoing process. Relapse is a hallmark of addictive disorders, and is the rule rather than the exception after a successful course of treatment. Thus, the likelihood of long-term maintenance of an abstinent lifestyle is enhanced by attention to relapse prevention. This four-stage treatment model implies that different therapeutic tasks will be appropriate at each stage. Importantly, although much attention is directed towards the components of active treatment, relatively little attention has been devoted to the tasks of engagement and persuasion.

Engagement

Voluntary engagement in treatment may take place if the client sees that affiliation with a treatment agency can be of benefit. Alternately, engagement may be coercive or involuntary, as in the case of referral from the criminal justice system or as a condition of discharge after an involuntary admission. As with substance abusing persons without schizophrenia, coerced involvement in substance abuse treatment may provide a window of opportunity to expose SSA clients to information about substance abuse.

In traditional treatment settings, dual diagnosis clients have poor outpatient attendance records and frequently drop out of treatment (e.g., Hall, Popkin, DeVaul, & Stickney, 1977). Even under the best of conditions, such difficulties can be expected. For example, in an outpatient therapy group designed specifically for persons with SSA, 66% of weekly group meetings were attended over the course of a year (Hellerstein & Meehan, 1987). Similarly, dually diagnosed participants who completed a social problem-solving treatment attended an average of two-thirds of the group sessions (Carey, Carey, & Meisler, 1990). Even in comprehensive programs specifically designed for dual diagnosis clients, drop out rates have been high (e.g., Kofoed, Kania, Walsh & Atkinson, 1986).

One can speculate about the many causes of poor attendance and attrition. Clients with SSA often lead chaotic lives, with many interruptions of a daily routine. The cognitive effects of coexisting disorders may result in poor planning and time management. They may be easily influenced by peers who devalue treatment attendance. They may avoid treatment when actively using substances, or when recovering from substance use. Normally occurring ambivalence about recovery may result in avoidance. Some clients may find it difficult to "fit in" to a treatment setting that does not acknowledge their unique lifestyle and problems.

In the four-stage model presented earlier, poor attendance and attrition reflect a problem with engagement. Convincing clients that treatment has something to offer them requires a clear idea of what they need and value. Incentives for participation in treatment may include help in obtaining food, housing, clothing, medications to relieve distressing symptoms, socialization or recreation opportunities, and avoidance of legal consequences (cf., Osher & Kofoed, 1989). An example of a minimal intervention designed to enhance attendance was reported by Carey and Carey (1990). In the context of a day treatment program for mentally ill chemical abusers, offering fast food coupons or free bowling passes contingent upon achieving a designated attendance criterion successfully increased the amount of time spent participating in the program. Other versions of continency management have been used in methadone maintenance and other drug treatment programs; this approach may be helpful in increasing exposure to treatment among clients with SSA.

Persuasion: Learning Why to Get Sober

Many clients who come to our attention are not ready for active treatment. Instead, they are not convinced that their substance use is a problem, and if it is, that abstinence is a necessary goal for them. Several approaches can be taken to persuade clients to change harmful substance abuse patterns.

Motivational interventions. These clients often enter treatment lacking "insight" into the source of their problems and "motivation" to change their substance use, just like their counterparts without schizophrenia. This combination, sometimes referred to as "denial," can be a source of great frustration to treatment providers. Recent reconceptualizations of "motivation" suggest that these frustrations result from inappropriate expectations on the part of treatment providers (Miller & Rollnick, 1991). Specifically, if motivation is viewed as a state of readiness for change, rather than a personality trait, then the task of the therapist is to help the client move to a greater readiness for change. Guidelines have been developed for enhancing this motivational state (Miller & Rollnick, 1991). Although not developed specifically for clients with SSA, these guidelines actually integrate approaches used by substance abuse and mental health professionals.

The principles of motivational intervention (Miller & Rollnick, 1991) overlap with the therapeutic tasks of the persuasion stage. These principles are: (a) express empathy, (b) develop discrepancy, (c) avoid argumentation, (d) roll with resistance, and (e) support self-efficacy. *Expressing empathy* involves nonjudgmental listening, acceptance of the whole client (including substance use and its problems), and acknowledgement that ambivalence about change is normal. *Developing discrepancy* refers to the process of highlighting the difference between the client's current behavior and his/her desired goals. Specific suggestions for developing discrepancy will be elaborated further below. *Avoiding argumentation* is consistent with recommendations to avoid confrontational approaches typical of more traditional substance abuse treatment approaches. Miller and Rollnick (1991) suggest that arguing with a client that a problem exists is likely to create psychological reactance — that is, the tendency to take the opposite position in order to assert one's freedom. In addition, clients with SSA are likely to have difficulty dealing with expressed emotion (Hooley, 1985), further reducing the effectiveness of a confrontational approach. *Rolling with the resistance* refers to the process of offering but not forcing new perspectives, and looking for opportunities to reframe or reinforce accurate perceptions. Encountering resistance is a signal to change tactics; optimally, the client will verbalize the problems he/she is having and the need to change. Finally, *supporting self-efficacy* refers to enhancing clients confidence in their ability to cope with the task of recovery. This is a significant area of vulnerability for many clients with schizophrenia. However, belief in the potential for change is an important prerequisite for motivation.

These principles can be applied to the treatment of persons with SSA. At any point in a substance abuser's career, an implicit cost-benefit ratio exists which determines whether or not the substance abuse will continue. During periods of active abuse, the perception of the benefits outweighs the costs. In other words, positive consequences of substance use (e.g., social facilitation, relief of anxiety or boredom) are more salient than the negative consequences (e.g., risk of psychotic decompensation, expense). Importantly, the abuser's perceptions (not objective reality) enter into the equation. When the ratio tips in favor of greater perceived costs than benefits, the stage is set for change. For this reason, hospitalization or other crises provide opportunities to talk about changing substance use patterns.

Clients sometimes come to acknowledge this changing balance on their own, and can verbalize the mounting costs and diminishing benefits (although rarely in those terms). In this case, the therapist's job is to reinforce the accuracy of client's perceptions and to channel that discomfort into active steps to diminish the costs of abuse and to enhance the benefits of abstinence.

However, for many clients who come to our attention, the ratio has not yet tipped; they do not yet see that the costs of continued abuse outweigh the benefits to them. As pointed out by Mueser et al. (1992), clients with schizophrenia may have particular difficulty in perceiving the consequences of continued use, due to cognitive limitations as well as a generally more impaired baseline of social and psychological functioning. In addition, they may not experience the typical losses (job, family, friends, reputation) that often motivate non-psychiatric clients to abstain. Again, the job of the therapist is to influence the perception of costs and benefits. Increasing awareness of costs can be done in several ways:

- Provide new information about problems that are abuse-related (e.g., liver dysfunction);

- Reframe past events, highlighting the role that alcohol or drug use played (e.g., in rehospitalization, loss of housing, family arguments);

- Provide feedback about changes in client's psychiatric state perceived by the therapist that appear to be resulting from, or exacerbated by, substance use;

- Engage in ongoing discussions of the role that substance use plays in the client's everyday life.

In general, the therapist attempts to identify the ways that substance use has hindered life goals important to the client. The therapist can also identify ways that substance use may be failing to provide the sought-after benefits, by pointing out the differences between short-term and long-term effects. For example, temporary relief of auditory hallucinations may be followed by an exacerbation once the drug intoxication wears off. Similarly, the feeling of belonging in a group may be contingent upon the client providing alcohol or marijuana, at great financial cost.

Enhancing awareness of the benefits of abstinence is also an important task for the therapist. Do not assume that the client can see these; many clients with schizophrenia do not expect good things to happen to them. Assistance in applying for decent housing, or for entry into a job training program, or access to greater sums of spending money are all examples of incentives that could be made contingent upon a certain criterion of abstinence. The challenge inherent in framing the benefits of abstinence is that most tangible benefits do not occur right away. They are long-term rewards, but we know that motivation is maximized by more frequent, short-term rewards. Therefore, the therapist should seek intermediate incentives for abstinence that will continue to motivate clients until they can realize the primary benefits of changing abuse patterns.

To summarize the relevance of motivational interviewing in the persuasion stage of treatment for clients with SSA: (a) It is nonconfrontational; (b) it views motivation for change as a dynamic state rather than a static trait; (c) readiness to change can be influenced by major life crises and by therapeutic intervention; (d) building readiness to change may be a long-term process; and (e) key elements include creating discrepancies, altering the perceived cost-benefit ratio, and enhancing self-efficacy.

Psychoeducational groups. Several authors have found psychoeducational groups to be useful in the treatment of persons with SSA (Carey 1989; Sciacca, 1987) Frequently, these clients lack accurate information about the nature of their illness, their medications, the effects of abused substances, and the interactions among them. Providing this information in an educational format is minimally threatening and potentially more engaging than formal "therapy," although more process-oriented formats have been explored (Kofoed & Keys, 1988).

If used as part of the persuasion stage of treatment, a commitment to abstinence is generally not required for group participation. However, one of the goals of the group might be to enhance the motivation for abstinence. Importantly, clients should not participate in groups or other treatment-related activities while under the influence of alcohol or illicit drugs.

The group leader might present information on a given topic, lead a discussion, and answer questions that arise. Short questionnaires, self-tests, and charts/diagrams are engaging and useful for stimulating discussion. The leader should reinforce information-seeking, as well as making appropriate cause-and-effect connections between psychiatric symptoms, substance use, and its consequences.

Psychoeducational groups tend not to be confrontational by design; however, as members volunteer their experiences relevant to topics, gentle social pressure is often brought to bear on members who do not acknowledge negative aspects of their substance use. Clients who are acutely psychotic are unlikely to benefit and may be disruptive even in a fairly structured group. Nonetheless, participation in a psychoeducational group may be an effective method of introducing many persons with SSA to concerns about their use of alcohol and/or drugs.

Active Treatment: Learning How to Get Sober

Once an interest is expressed in reducing substance use or in eliminating the negative consequences of substance use (i.e., one has learned *why* to be sober), the task is to learn *how* to be sober. During the active treatment phase, a combination of individual counseling and group modalities is recommended.

Individual counseling. The ongoing relationship with a treatment provider necessitated by the presence of major mental illness provides an excellent method of monitoring and encouraging recovery efforts. Whether or not the primary treatment provider also conducts the substance abuse treatment, he/she ought to thoroughly integrate assessment of substance use, its relationship to psychiatric symptoms, and its consequences into mental health treatment. It is all too common for a mental health professional to ignore substance use issues with the justification, "I am not treating him/her for *that.*" However, our clients must understand that substance use is relevant to their psychiatric condition; they must also believe that therapists and doctors are allies in the very difficult task of overcoming dual disabilities. In addition, individual counseling may be the only acceptable method of exposure to active treatment for clients with SSA who are not comfortable in groups.

Psychoeducational groups. Group therapies represent well-established modalities of active treatment for both schizophrenia and substance abuse (Kaplan & Sadock, 1982). As a continuation from the previous phase, the psychoeducational approach helps clients to understand what to expect from the recovery process. The similarities among acute withdrawal symptoms, extended withdrawal discomfort, and symptoms of mental illness can be confusing for clients. The ubiquity of cravings for drugs/alcohol, anxiety, depression, and self-doubt during recovery are also relevant topics. The distinctions between "good" drugs (i.e., prescribed medications), and "bad" drugs (i.e., alcohol and illicit drugs) can be challenging and bears frequent repetition. Experience with clients with SSA suggests that information must be repeated often to ensure adequate comprehension and retention. This format can develop into a social support group for recovering clients, and successful role models can be identified as a means of boosting the self-efficacy of struggling clients.

Coping skills training. Developing the skills needed to cope with ongoing stressors and to maintain an abstinent lifestyle poses a major challenge for a person with SSA. In many cases, alcohol or drug use has served important coping functions. Perhaps substance use has served as a social facilitator, or a way of dealing with uncomfortable emotions, or as a source of an "image" preferable to that of "mental patient." In order to successfully abstain, the client with SSA has to cope with these needs in other ways. Given ample evidence of social and emotional deficits associated with schizophrenia (Nuechterlein & Dawson, 1984b), it is clear that learning how to be sober involves the learning of a variety of coping skills.

Many clients with SSA find that they are comfortable with people only when high; the superficial relationships developed around using drugs provide a social network with mimimal intimacy demands; alternatively, these clients may find acceptance from an "outgroup" of substance abusers which is not readily obtained by mainstream society. Thus, promising areas for coping skills training include conversational, assertive, and other social skills, to maximize the chance that the recovering person with SSA can obtain social support necessary to facilitate recovery and to learn how to relate to people without having to use alcohol or drugs. Medication management and relapse management skills will be needed in order to lessen the reliance on illicit drugs to manage uncomfortable symptoms. In addition, many clients also will benefit from instruction and "consumer" skill development related to obtaining needed services from understaffed mental health (and other) service systems.

Individuals with schizophrenia may have difficulty translating new knowledge into behavior change. For this reason, the skills training model provides clear guidelines for making this translation. Specifically, skills training provides structure in the form of (a) definition of skills to be learned, (b) modeling of those skills by group leaders, (c) rehearsal of skills in session and practice out of session, and (d) corrective feedback on implementation of skills. The ultimate goal of skills training is to empower clients to be more effective in their social roles.

Lifestyle modification. It can be difficult to appreciate what a comprehensive lifestyle change we ask of recovering persons. Use of alcohol and drugs becomes a primary leisure time activity, structures an otherwise unstructured existence, provides an identity, and usually results in a social network composed primarily of other substance users. It is common (and appropriate) to advise the recovering person to avoid the people, places, and things associated with substance use; this advice, which is theoretically sound in terms of avoiding triggers for use, reduces what may already be a meager social network. However, clients with SSA have a low probability of establishing an abstinent lifestyle if they continue to frequent familiar people and places. If we cannot help our clients to generate alternatives, change may not occur. Therefore, some assistance in structuring time, and in providing drug-free leisure/recreational activities should be incorporated into the active treatment phase. Lifestyle modification includes changing how and where people eat and drink, where and with whom they spend their time, where and with whom they live. Although these concerns may be seen as the luxury of only comprehensive treatment programs, they may be essential to the success of active treatment efforts. If contact time is limited, allocate your efforts to this therapeutic task before investing in other (more typical) tasks, such as exploring the developmental precipitants of the substance abuse problem.

Relapse Prevention: Maintaining An Abstinent Lifestyle

Both schizophrenia and substance abuse are disorders for which relapse is to be anticipated. Many persons with schizophenia experience periodic exacerbation of symptoms, and, for the majority of substance abusers, recovery consists of periods of abstinence interrupted by the resumption of drinking or drug use. Thus, therapy targeted at prevention and management of relapses should be incorporated into every psychosocial intervention for persons with SSA. Because substance use frequently exacerbates psychiatric symptoms, and psychiatric decompensation often triggers substance use due to poor judgment or an effort to manage symptoms, relapse prevention should address both types of relapse simultaneously. Importantly, a relapse or slip should not be viewed as a failure, but rather as helpful feedback regarding areas of vulnerability and inadequacy of existing coping skills. Just as with other mental disorders (and life challenges), we strive for effective *management* rather than complete *cure*. Fortunately, the principles and strategies of relapse prevention are well-described (e.g., Marlatt & Gordon, 1985), and they can be enacted in both group and individual formats.

Relapse prevention groups provide social support for ongoing efforts to maintain abstinence, as well as the opportunity to learn from others' successes and failures. Therapeutic activities include identification of common relapse situations, and development of coping strategies to minimize the risk of relapse. Group members can help each other practice coping skills, using principles of modeling, rehearsal and performance feedback. In addition, once slips occur, group problem-solving and social support may serve to boost self-efficacy and minimize the consequences of a slip.

Some persons with SSA may not be comfortable in group settings, and relapse prevention can be conducted on an individual level. With the client's participation, social or psychological situations that increase the risk for decompensation and/or substance use can be identified, and "plans of action" can be developed. A therapist can tailor this analysis to clients' capacity for self-understanding, and their unique strengths and weaknesses. The results of exposure to "high risk" situations can be discussed.

Consistent with this view of relapse, appropriate response to lapses include prompt reinvolvement in treatment, review of psychiatric status and medication needs, and enhancement of support systems. Staff can reinforce the return to treatment after a relapse, and credit the client for taking responsible action if he/she seeks help. Given the likelihood of relapse in this population, appropriate therapeutic goals include longer abstinent periods, shorter durations of relapse to substance use, and management of acute exacerbations of schizophrenic symptoms without resorting to substance use. Thus, in lieu of extended abstinent and symptom-free periods, measure therapeutic success in terms of change in the frequency and duration of relapses, as well as overall improvement of function.

Self-Help Groups

Most substance abuse treatment programs recommend participation in self-help groups such as Alcoholics Anonymous (AA) and Narcotics Anonymous (NA). However, for reasons related to psychiatric symptomatology (e.g., paranoid thinking, social discomfort, unusual behaviors) and unrelated to motivation for treatment, self-help groups may not be therapeutic for all persons with SSA. Thus, participation in self-help groups can be encouraged but not required.

Self-help groups can provide a very real service to these clients. By their nature they follow a familiar structure. Many groups readily accept "drop-ins" and allow passive participation. In most communities, AA/NA groups take place regularly, sometimes several times a day, providing a social structure at times when psychiatric treatment may not be available. Furthermore, self-help groups utilize concrete and easily remembered slogans, such as "One day at a time," which are repeated often. These slogans facilitate communication among individuals whose cognitive processing may be compromised.

Attempts to integrate clients with SSA into self-help groups have run into difficulties. Some AA/NA groups are more tolerant of mentally ill participants than others. Traditionally, the self-help community has distrusted psychiatric treatment, even discouraging its members from using psychiatric medications in an effort to achieve a fully drug-free recovery. However, AA now publishes literature that explicitly supports the need for some of its members to take psychiatric medications. Clients with SSA may also have difficulty obtaining a sponsor, due to social skills deficits or lack of willing candidates. Since each AA/NA group has a "personality" of its own, clients with SSA should be encouraged to visit other meetings if their first experiences have not been welcoming. Another option is to elicit support from local AA/NA organizers to start a new meeting for those with dual diagnoses. Several treatment programs have reported success in establishing and maintaining such "double trouble" groups (e.g., Carey, 1989).

Family Education/Support

Treatment guidelines for both substance abuse and schizophrenia recommend eliciting support from family members and involving them in treatment. However, family support may not be readily available to persons with SSA, many of whom have alienated family members and live isolated lives. When family connections are desired, family members frequently need information about the dual disorders. They also need help in discriminating what is appropriate support of their relative versus what is inappropriate enabling of dysfunctional behavior. Questions often arise regarding how to set limits on substance use behaviors and how to enforce agreed-upon consequences. Many families are reluctant to set limits for fear of provoking a relapse or placing their relative at risk in some way. More basic questions arise regarding what kind of behaviors to expect from the mental illness, and what symptoms might be more directly related to substance use. By empowering the family with information and support for their difficult task, they help to generalize treatment principles outside of the treatment setting.

SPECIAL TREATMENT ISSUES

Several additional treatment issues warrant further discussion. Some, such as cultural considerations in the treatment process, HIV/AIDS risk, and the interface of the mental health with other social service systems, will be covered in other chapters. Three concerns of particular relevance to persons with SSA deserve focus: (a) the potential impact of cognitive dysfunction, (b) the revolving door problem, and (c) the need for a longitudinal perspective on treatment.

Cognitive Dysfunction

A major factor limiting the effectiveness of treatment may be the degree of neuropsychological or cognitive impairment experienced by dual diagnosis clients. As many as two-thirds of alcoholics entering treatment exhibit measurable cognitive impairment (Meek, Clark, & Solana, 1989). Alcohol-related cognitive deficits include impaired memory, problem-solving, abstraction abilities and perceptual-motor skills (Chelune & Parker, 1981). Although many aspects of cognitive function do recover with cessation of drinking, measurable impairment has been observed even after extended abstinence. Abuse of other central nervous system depressants and cocaine also contribute to cognitive dysfunction (Grant, Adams, Carlin, Rennick, Judd & Schoof, 1978; O'Malley & Gawin, 1990). Cognitive impairment has been associated with failure to remember the content of treatment sessions (Sanchez-Craig & Walker, 1982), and with quicker relapses (Gregson & Taylor, 1977).

Cognitive impairments, especially attention, memory, and information processing deficits, are characteristic of both acute and residual stages of schizophrenia (Nuechterlein & Dawson, 1984a). As with substance abusers, cognitive dysfunction limits the ability of clients to benefit from treatment. For example, memory deficits in persons with schizophrenia predict poorer treatment outcomes (Mueser, Bellack, Douglas, & Wade, 1991). Given that clients with schizophrenia exhibit cognitive impairment in the absence of substance abuse, it is important to determine whether these cognitive difficulties are exacerbated by the acute and/or chronic effects of substance abuse. It is possible that clients with SSA are even more sensitive to drug-related cognitive impairment because of their coexisting mental illness, and/or their use of psychiatric medications. Meek and colleagues (1989) point out that staff interpretation of, and response to difficult behaviors can be influenced by information regarding the existence of cognitive deficits. Recommendations include:

- Use clear and unambiguous rules;

- Communicate behavioral expectations clearly and simply;

- Err on the side of giving directions rather than relying on client-generated insights;

- Focus on concrete, short-term goals;

- Repeat important educational information and therapeutic themes;

- Check for comprehension and retention;

- Insist on translation of talk into behavior; e.g., use behavioral rehearsal;

- Refer for neuropsychological evaluation when cognitive function is questionned.

Current psychosocial treatments for both severe mental illness and substance abuse disorders emphasize psychoeducation and coping skills training (e.g., Liberman, Mueser, & DeRisi, 1989; Monti, Abrams, Kadden, & Cooney, 1989). These treatment components makes substantial demands on attention, concentration, memory, learning, and problem-solving abilities. Systematic evaluations of the combined effects of substance abuse and schizophrenia on cognitive functioning are needed in order to optimally adapt existing and to develop new treatments.

The Revolving Door Problem

Clients with SSA use costly inpatient services more frequently than clients without substance abuse problems (Bartels, Teague, Drake, Clark, Bush & Noordsy, 1993), although their admissions tend to be of shorter duration (Safer, 1987). Often the cause of this revolving door problem is the acute exacerbation of symptoms due to substance use, and the quick resolution of the crisis following the elimination of the abused substances. Inpatient staff no longer see a need for hospitalization, and they respond to the client's wishes to be discharged once stabilized. In times of diminishing resources, this costly pattern of service utilization is understandable but also potentially self-defeating. One way of minimizing the revolving door pattern is to acknowledge the cause of the crisis (i.e., substance use) and to address the frequent lack of coordination between inpatient and outpatient services as well as between mental health and substance abuse services.

Studies indicate that dual diagnosis clients are less likely to be referred to alcohol/drug treatment and they are less likely to follow through with referrals when they are made (Solomon & Davis, 1986). Part of the problem may be the absence of treatment programs that will accept mentally ill persons with substance abuse. Few communities possess a comprehensive treatment program as described in this chapter, and many mental health professionals report that existing substance abuse programs restrict access to their clients with schizophrenia. However, even in the absence of specialized programs, several steps can be taken within the mental health system to maximize the usefulness of inpatient admissions and to better coordinate inpatient and outpatient services.

- Use of urine screens upon admission is recommended for suspected or confirmed substance abuse. This procedure is standard for substance abuse treatment, yet not always employed in mental health settings. The results of urine screens can be used to document symptom exacerbations that are related to recent substance use. Crises precipitated by intoxication, withdrawal, or the social consequences of substance use (i.e., loss of housing, lack of money, family disputes) can be used as "windows of opportunity" to help the client with SSA reevaluate the current cost-benefit ratio of continuing to use substances. The situationally induced motivation to change can be channeled by having the client speak with outpatient treatment staff while still an inpatient, and by engaging the client's support system (spouse, parents, residential staff) in contracted agreements covering future acceptable behavior regarding substance use.

• Communication with the outpatient service who will be taking responsibility for the client before the discharge is even more essential when substance abuse is involved. Discharging a recently detoxified client back to an environment saturated with drug use cues, or to an unstructured daily routine, or to a wait of weeks before a therapist or counselor can be seen will result in loss of all gains achieved. Thus, to the extent possible, follow-up services for client with SSA should be in place before discharge.

• Extended inpatient stays may be useful as a means of achieving a stable, drug-free state for evaluation of clients with SSA. Thus, maintaining a client with SSA in the hospital after the acute crisis abates may be justified for several reasons. This period can be used to observe functional abilities when abstinent, to adjust medications, and to attempt to engage in treatment in the absence of powerful drug use cues.

The motivations and needs for the use of inpatient services by clients with SSA vary, and the optimal use of limited treatment resources cannot be dictated without knowledge of an individual client. However, better communication among treatment providers, and willingness to accommodate to the needs generated by coexisting disorders should reduce the risk of the revolving door phenomenon.

A Longitudinal Perspective

The combination of chronic, relapsing disorders, managed primarily on an outpatient basis, suggests that change will be a long-term process. Treatment providers should see their role as shaping the attitudes and skills necessary to reduce the impact of substance use on clients' lives. This approach is necessary for at least two reasons. First, substance abusers (with and without schizophrenia) evolve in their readiness to change. Critical incidents can move individuals through stages of change; although critical incidents may be created through contact with treatment providers, the most powerful motivators of change often occur spontaneously in relationships and through personal growth experiences. Recovering persons often relate a point in their lives when they become "sick and tired of being sick and tired;" at that point, and not before, they will participate actively and sincerely in treatment. There is no reason to believe that this process differs in clients with SSA. Second, the process of difficult therapeutic change is supported by a person's personal resources and environment. Clients with SSA may have fewer psychological coping skills to deal with the stress of change; they usually have fewer social supports and less supportive physical environments. As a result, "momentum" established within treatment frequently dissipates when the client walks out the door. Add these circumstances to the lack of consistent and comprehensive services for dually diagnosed persons, and the result is slow and unsteady progress at best.

Progress can be made, however! Treatment providers would be advised to do the following:

- Cultivate patience, and the ability to recognize small changes in the desired direction;

- Attend to naturally occurring changes in substance use patterns and offer your perceptions of the impact of substance use on their functioning;

- Avoid negative judgments about the person, but set and enforce limits on behaviors;

- Look for opportunities to engage in motivational interventions;

- Respond promptly to interest in active treatment, either within your own treatment plan or by referral;

- Offer assistance and strong advocacy contingent upon behavioral evidence of efforts to reduce or eliminate substance abuse;

- Expect periodic breaks in treatment contact, and engage in active outreach to reduce their duration and frequency;

- Provide efficacy-enhancing feedback when, for whatever reasons, the client demonstrates an ability to control or reduce substance use.

Experience suggests that, over time, the development of a collaborative relationship, the consistency of informational feedback, and the establishment of a social network supportive of abstinence will result in greater receptiveness to changing substance abuse patterns.

CONCLUSION

The treatment of substance abuse in persons with schizophrenia is a task requiring creativity and teamwork. However, the rewards can also be great. Clients become frustrated with fragmented services, and with treatment professionals who neglect to ask about important aspects of their functioning. Once substance use is integrated into a complete clinical picture, many clients express relief at the prospects of making sense out of a confusing set of experiences. For their welfare and our own, we must accept that challenge.

REFERENCES

Ban, T.A. (1977). Alcoholism and schizophrenia: Diagnostic and therapeutic considerations. *Alcohol: Clinical and Experimental Research. 1*, 113–117.

Banys, P. (1988). The clinical use of disulfiram (Antabuse): A review. *Journal of Psychoactive Drugs. 20*, 243–261.

Bartels, S.J., Teague, G.B., Drake, R.E., Clark, R.E., Bush, P.W., & Noordsy, D.L. (1993). Substance abuse in schizophrenia: Service utilization and costs. *Journal of Nervous and Mental Disease. 181*, 227–232.

Carey, K.B. (1989). Treatment of the mentally ill chemical abuser: Description of the Hutchings day treatment program. *Psychiatric Quarterly. 60*, 303–316.

Carey, K.B., & Carey, M.P. (1990). Enhancing the treatment attendance of mentally ill chemical abusers. *Journal of Behavior Therapy and Experimental Psychiatry. 21*, 205–209.

Carey, M.P., Carey, K.B., & Meisler, A.W. (1990). Training mentally ill chemical abusers in social problem solving. *Behavior Therapy. 21*, 511–518.

Chelune, G.J., & Parker, J.B. (1981). Neuropsychological deficits associated with chronic alcohol abuse. *Clinical Psychology Review. 1*, 181–195.

Dixon, L., Haas, G., Weiden, P., Sweeney, J., & Frances, A. (1990). Acute effects of drug abuse in schizophrenic patients: Clinical observations and patients' self-reports. *Schizophrenia Bulletin, 16*, 69–79.

Drake, R.E., Osher, F.C., & Wallace, M.A. (1989). Alcohol use and abuse in schizophrenia: A prospective community study. *Journal of Nervous and Mental Disease, 177*, 408–414.

Grant, I., Adams, K.M., Carlin, A.S., Rennick, P.M., Judd, L.L., & Schoof, K. (1978). The collaborative neuropsychological study of polydrug users. *Archives of General Psychiatry. 35*, 1063–1074.

Gregson, R.A.M., & Taylor, G.M. (1977). Prediction of relapse in men alcoholics. *Journal of Studies on Alcohol. 38*, 1749–1760.

Hall, R.C.W., Popkin, M.K., DeVaul, R., & Stickney, S.K. (1977). The effect of unrecognized drug abuse on diagnosis and therapeutic outcome. *American Journal of Drug and Alcohol Abuse. 4*, 455–465.

Heinrichs, R.W. (1993). Schizophrenia and the brain. *American Psychiatry, 48*, 221–233.

Hellerstein, D.J., & Meehan, B. (1987). Outpatient group therapy for schizophrenic substance abusers. *American Journal of Psychiatry, 144*, 1337–1339.

Hooley, J. (1985). Expressed emotion: A review of the critical literature. *Clinical Psychology Review. 5*, 119–140.

Kaplan, H.I., & Sadock, B.J. (1982). *Comprehensive group psychotherapy*, 2nd Ed. Baltimore: Williams & Wilkins.

Kofoed, L., Kania, J., Walsh, T., & Atkinson, R.M. (1986). Outpatient treatment of patients with substance abuse and coexisting psychiatric disorder. *American Journal of Psychiatry. 143*, 867–872.

Kofoed, L., & Keys, A. (1988). Using group therapy to persuade dual-diagnosis patients to seek substance abuse treatment. *Hospital and Community Psychiatry, 39*, 1201–1211.

Liberman, R.P., Mueser, K.T., & DeRisi, W.J. (1989). *Social skills training for psychiatric patients*. Elmsford, NY: Pergamon.

Marlatt, G.A., & Gordon, J.R. (1985). *Relapse prevention: Maintenance strategies in the treatment of addictive behaviors*. New York: Guilford.

Meek, P.S., Clark, H.W., & Solana, V.L. (1989). Neurocognitive impairment: The unrecognized component of dual diagnosis in substance abuse treatment. *Journal of Psychoactive Drugs. 21*, 153–160.

Miller, W.M., & Rollnick, S. (1991). *Motivational interviewing: Preparing people to change addictive behavior*. New York: Guilford.

Monti, P.M., Abrams, D.B., Kadden, R.M., & Cooney, N.L. (1989). *Treating alcohol dependence*. New York: Guilford.

Mueser, K.T., Bellack, A.S., & Blanchard, J.J. (1992). Comorbidity of schizophrenia and substance abuse: Implications for treatment. *Journal of Consulting and Clinical Psychology. 60*, 845–856.

Mueser, K.T., Bellack, A.S., Douglas, M.S., & Wade, J.H. (1991). Prediction of social skill acquisition in schizophrenic and major affective disorder patients from memory and symptomatology. *Psychiatry Research. 37*, 281–296.

Mueser, K.T., Yarnold, P.R., Levinson, D.F., Singh, H., Bellack, A.S., Kee, K., Morrison, R.L., & Yadalam, K.G. (1990). Prevalence of substance abuse in schizophrenia: Demographic and clinical correlates. *Schizophrenia Bulletin. 16*, 31–56.

Nuechterlein, K.H., & Dawson, M.E. (1984-a). Information processing and attentional functioning in the developmental course of schizophrenic disorders. *Schizophrenia Bulletin. 10*, 160–203.

Nuechterlein, K.H., & Dawson, M.E. (1984-b). A heuristic vulnerability/stress model of schizophrenic episodes. *Schizophrenia Bulletin. 10*, 300–312.

O'Malley, S.S., & Gawin, F.H. (1990). Abstinence symptomatology and neuropsychological impairment in chronic cocaine abusers. In J.W. Spence & J.J. Boren (Eds.), *Residual effects of abused drugs on behavior* (National Institute on Drug Abuse Research Monograph No. 101, pp. 179–190). Washington, DC: National Institute on Drug Abuse.

Osher, F.C., & Kofoed, L.L. (1989). Treatment of patients with psychiatric and psychoactive substance abuse disorders. *Hospital and Community Psychiatry. 40*, 1025–1030.

Pristach, C.A., & Smith, C.M. (1990). Medication compliance and substance abuse among schizophrenic patients. *Hospital and Community Psychiatry. 41*, 1345–1348.

Regier, D.A., Farmer, M.E., Rae, D.S., Locke, B.Z., Keith, S.J., Judd, L.L., & Goodwin, F.K. (1990). Comorbidity of mental disorders with alcohol and other drug abuse. *Journal of the American Medical Association. 264*, 2511–2518.

Safer, D.J. (1987). Substance abuse by young adult chronic patients. *Hospital and Community Psychiatry. 38*, 511–514.

Sanchez-Craig, M., & Walker, K. (1982). Teaching coping skills to chronic alcoholics in a coeducational halfway house: I. Assessment of programme effects. *British Journal of Addiction, 77*, 35–50.

Sciacca, K. (1987). New initiatives in the treatment of the chronic patient with alcohol/substance abuse problems. *Tie Lines*, IC (July), 5–6.

Siris, S.G. (1990). Pharmacological treatment of substance-abusing schizophrenic patients. *Hospital and Community Psychiatry. 16*, 111–122.

Solomon, P., & Davis, J.M. (1986). The effects of alcohol abuse among the new chronically mentally ill. *Social Work in Health Care. 11*, 65–74.

NOTES

I gratefully acknowledge the patients and staff of Richard H. Hutchings Psychiatric Center for their assistance in my search for understanding. Preparation of this chapter was supported in part by National Institute on Drug Abuse Grant DA07635.

7

Mood Disorders and
Substance Use

ROGER D. WEISS and EILEEN J. WONG

Treating a patient with coexisting mood and substance use disorders poses a number of serious challenges for clinicians. First, these patients may exhibit a wide variety of symptoms, thus potentially presenting great diagnostic difficulties. Moreover, the treatment of this patient population is complicated by the fact that each of these disorders may alter the course and worsen the prognosis of the other, including increasing the risk of suicide. Fortunately, recent research and clinical experience has led to an increasing body of knowledge focusing on the evaluation and treatment of this heterogeneous group of patients.

PATTERNS OF CO-OCCURRENCE

Epidemiologic studies have highlighted the frequent pattern of co-occurrence of substance abuse and mood disorders. The ECA study (Regier et al., 1990) confirmed the finding of earlier clinical studies that substance abuse occurs in patients with primary mood disorders at a higher prevalance rate than in the general population. Indeed, the frequency of substance use disorders among patients with mood disorders was twice that of the general population, with approximately one-third of those in the mood disorder group reporting substance dependence. Interestingly, substance abuse among patients with bipolar disorder was far more prevalent than among patients with unipolar depression, with prevalance rates of 56.1% and 27.2% respectively. Strikingly, the probability of drug use other than alcohol in patients with bipolar I disorder was eleven-fold greater than that of the general population.

The ECA study also confirmed the higher prevalence rate of mood disorders among primary substance abusers when compared to the rest of the community; mood disorders were almost twice as likely in patients with alcohol disorders and almost five times more prevalent in the drug dependent group. Again, the association of substance use disorders and bipolar disorder was particularly strong; the probability that a patient with a primary alcohol diagnosis would also have bipolar disorder or unipolar depression was 5.1 and 1.3 times greater than that in the general population, respectively.

Although it has long been recognized that there is a greater than expected rate of substance use disorders among patients with mood disorders, this mere coexistence does not explain the cause of the association. Why, then, do patients with unipolar or bipolar illness abuse drugs more often than other individuals?

One frequently cited hypothesis for the use and abuse of psychoactive drugs in general is the self-medication theory (Khantzian, 1985), which states that patients use specific drugs in order to alleviate intolerable mood states. The self-medication hypothesis has been criticized because it has been largely based on anecdotal data gathered from relatively small groups of persons with substance abuse who were in psychotherapy. However, recent empirical studies examining the self-medication hypothesis have shed further light on its strengths and limitations. In particular, we recently examined the self-medication hypothesis for depression by asking a group of 494 hospitalized drug dependent patients about their reasons for drug use, and the effects of their drug use (Weiss, Griffin & Mirin, 1992-b). We found that 63% of drug dependent patients claimed to use drugs when depressed, and that 68% found that drug use improved their mood. Interestingly, the likelihood of relief of mood symptoms was not related to drug of choice or to the presence or absence of a diagnosis of major depression.

Although it has been shown that retrospective self-reports of drug effects often conflict with observational data, patients use drugs or alcohol because of their own perception of how they believe the drug will make them feel; the fact that others may dispute their perception does not necessarily change their own beliefs regarding how the drug will make them feel. Moreover, it is possible that even a brief period of mood elevation may be sufficient reason for a depressed patient to use drugs, even if this is followed by a succession of adverse consequences, including a worsening of mood. Indeed, some authors have speculated that mood change, rather than mood elevation, may be a primary motivator of drug use, particularly in depressed patients (Khantzian, 1989). As one patient stated, "I don't care what the long-term consequences are of my drinking. I know that I'll feel worse tomorrow, and I may even feel worse later tonight. But when I drink, I know that an hour later, I won't feel the way that I do when I start drinking, and that's all I care about."

Patients with bipolar or cyclothymic disorder may abuse substances for a variety of reasons. Some patients with these illnesses may attempt to relieve symptoms during the depressed phase of their illness, although patients with bipolar disorder are at higher risk to relapse during a period of hypomania than while depressed (Gawin & Kleber, 1986). Patients who are hypomanic or manic may use alcohol or drugs for a number of reasons. Some patients may wish to reduce unwanted symptoms of agitation, irritability, and insomnia; irritability is often cited as the primary manic symptom that leads to substance use. The use of certain drugs may also enhance more desirable symptoms of euphoria, grandiosity and hypersexuality. Our group and others have reported that a sizable group of patients with cocaine abuse and bipolar disorder or cyclothymia report use during the hypomanic phase in order to enhance their endogenously euphoric state (Gawin & Kleber 1986; Weiss, Mirin, Griffin & Michael, 1988). Contrary to certain epidemiologic studies (see Chapter 2), our clinical experience has led us to posit that treatment-seeking patients with euphoric mania tend to prefer stimulant drugs, which enhance their desirable endogenous symptoms. On the other hand, patients whose mania is characterized by primarily dysphoric symptoms tend to prefer alcohol, sedative-hypnotic drugs, marijuana, or opioids in an attempt to reduce these unwanted symptoms.

In addition to the potential direct reinforcing effects of substances of abuse in patients with primary mood disorders, depression or mania may interfere with an individual's ability to recognize the adverse consequences of drug use. Moreover, even individuals who may recognize the potentially harmful outcomes associated with their substance use may have particular difficulty conforming their behavior to stopping their substance use. For example, patients with hypomania are frequently grandiose and reckless, and often exercise poor judgment. Patients with these characteristics obviously will have a more difficult time either carefully considering the potential adverse consequences of their substance use or stopping themselves even if they conclude that this behavior will be ultimately harmful to them.

Depressed patients, particularly individuals with more severe forms of the disorder, are also at increased risk for substance use because of the effect of their mood on their thought processes and behavior. For example, hopelessness may lead a profoundly depressed patient to respond apathetically when considering the possibility of future drug-related problems. As one severely depressed patient said, "So my drinking is going to make my life miserable? So what?" For such patients, substance use offers a change in mood state, however brief, and an escape from reality for the duration of the period of intoxication. In such patients, the eventual consequences of their substance use, however grave, are often approached fearlessly. This is not to say that these patients are necessarily "in denial." Rather, many of these patients understand quite clearly that they are alcoholic, and that further drinking will lead to loss of control, adverse consequences, and the usual panoply of problems seen in patients with substance use disorders. However, these patients may be hopeless enough about the prospect of mood improvement that they simply do not care about the extra troubles that their substance use will probably cause.

Finally, a discussion of the co-occurrence of substance use disorders and mood disorders would be incomplete without highlighting the high rate of suicide in this population. Indeed, suicide rates of up to 15% have been cited among substance abusers (Marzuk & Mann, 1988; Schuckit, 1989). Some authors have speculated that this figure may in fact be an underestimate, since it does not include substance abuse-related injuries or deaths that are not clearly suicide attempts. While it is well known that depression increases the risk of suicide, the coexistence of a mood disorder and substance abuse clearly increases the lethality of either disorder, since substance use can lead to disinhibition, aggressiveness, poor judgment, incoordination, accident proneness, and an exacerbation of depressive, anxious, or psychotic symptoms that may all help to convert vague suicidal ideas into lethal actions.

SPECIAL DIAGNOSTIC ISSUES

Making the diagnosis of a mood disorder in a substance abusing person is frequently a very complex process. In the initial clinical interview, patients may be either intoxicated or withdrawing, and may thus be unable to provide a comprehensive history. Even if this is not the case, patients may present with a relatively vague chief complaint, and may be reluctant to share information either on the presence or extent of their active substance use, or the level of mood disturbance. Even in patients who are forthcoming, the accuracy of their recall may be limited. Moreover, studies by our group and others have shown that although addicted patients often give relatively accurate substance use histories, their recall of the temporal sequence of psychiatric symptoms and substance abuse tends to be quite unreliable (Rounsaville & Kleber, 1984; Weiss, Mirin & Griffin, 1992-a).

Even in the best of circumstances, i.e., cooperative patients with a solid memory who are forthcoming about their substance use and their mood disturbance, patients may present with a constellation of mood and behavioral disturbances that create a diagnostic dilemma. Indeed, obtaining pertinent medical and psychiatric history may further complicate the assessment. The clinical cases described below exemplify the types of diagnostic problems that may occur in such patients.

Ms. A, a 31-year old woman, was hospitalized with a diagnosis of cocaine and heroin dependence of seven years duration. Ms. A was diagnosed as having possible attention deficit disorder in childhood, and experienced a severe head injury in an automobile accident four years prior to admission. Following detoxification, she experienced severe craving for both cocaine and heroin, and frequently sought medications in a frenetic manner on the hospital unit. Her affect and mood were labile, ranging from anergic depression to a state of agitation with rapid, somewhat pressured speech.

Mr. B, a 50-year old man, was admitted because of a 25-year history of alcohol dependence. The patient was diagnosed with post-traumatic stress disorder secondary to war traumas, and had made several suicide attempts in the past, primarily when intoxicated with alcohol. His medical history was significant, due to the presence of congestive heart failure and adult onset diabetes mellitus. At admission, he complained of ongoing severe anxiety and depression, although it was unclear to him what the relationship was between these symptoms and his drinking, since he reported that "I'm always anxious, I'm always depressed, and I'm always drinking." His longest period of abstinence in the past several years was 10 days. Several days following his detoxification, he was apathetic and appeared unmotivated to participate in treatment. He complained of global insomnia and mild suicidal ideation.

These two cases reveal the potential complexity of the diagnostic process in evaluating patients with substance use disorders and coexisting mood disorders.

The major initial challenge that clinicians face in working with these patients involves determining the basis for their mood disturbances. In many cases, abnormal mood may be due to substance use, Axis I or Axis II psychiatric disorders other than mood disorders, and/or coexisting medical conditions. Indeed, Jaffe and Ciraulo (1986) have listed potential causes of depressive symptoms in alcoholic patients. These include direct and indirect toxic effects of alcohol, withdrawal, head trauma, social losses, other Axis I disorders (e.g., eating disorders or post-traumatic stress disorder), and personality disorders (e.g., borderline or narcissistic personality disorders). Moreover, these causes frequently interact to exacerbate depressive symptoms. Medical causes of depression must also be considered in such patients; it is possible, for example, that Mr. B's congestive heart failure and/or diabetes may have contributed to his psychiatric symptoms.

One physical condition of particular importance in patients with substance use disorders is human immunodeficiency virus (HIV) infection, which may present with a wide variety of disturbances of mood and/or cognition; needle-sharing, unprotected sex practices (due to disinhibited behavior), and/or the immunosuppressive effects of various drugs of abuse place this population at a higher risk for HIV-related disease. Considering the wide range of conditions that may contribute to mood symptoms, it is not surprising that clinical presentations of depression or hypomania in such patients are often atypical. Indeed, when several such factors coexist, the resultant symptoms may not meet the classical diagnostic criteria for mood disorders. Rather, the patient may appear to have either a subclinical or atypical form of a mood disorder.

How, then, can the clinician distinguish an alcohol or drug related mood syndrome from an autonomous mood disorder? Obtaining past history can sometimes be helpful; however, as we mentioned above, this may be vague and inaccurate. Moreover, patients' attitudes toward their substance use disorder may affect their recollection of their psychiatric history. For example, patients who believe that they drink in order to relieve their depression may state during an initial interview that they have been depressed even when alcohol-free. However, if such patients enter treatment, they may attend Alcoholics Anonymous (AA) meetings in which group members challenge their version of events and tell them that they are depressed *because* they drink. If they are convinced by the AA members of this new version of events, they may change their view of their history. In such cases, they may later state that their depression only occurred in the context of heavy drinking. Such a change can occur quite easily in patients who do not clearly recall the relationship between their drinking and their depression. Thus, patients' attitudes toward their drinking and their depression may color their history. For this reason, it is generally preferable not to make a firm diagnostic decision based on a single interview, particularly during early abstinence, when patients tend to be most confused and most subject to attitudinal shifts. Rather, a series of longitudinal interviews can help to distinguish between substance-related mood changes and autonomous mood disorders (see also Chapter 11).

There is some controversy regarding the length of time that a patient needs to be abstinent before an independent mood disorder can be diagnosed. Some authors, such as Schuckit (1985), have argued that a period of abstinence ranging up to 3 months is necessary before major depression can be diagnosed, whereas other researchers, notably Rounsaville, Anton, Carroll, Budde, Prusoff and Gawin (1991), have claimed that major depression can be diagnosed even during periods of active substance use, as long as the level of use has remained constant over a long period of time. Many other authors have argued intermediate views. Although this issue has not yet clearly been resolved, it is important to realize that withdrawal symptoms from different drugs of abuse are not all similar. Cocaine withdrawal, opioid withdrawal, and alcohol withdrawal all have distinctive sets of symptoms, and should not be confused with each other. Therefore, the differential diagnostic picture will vary, based on the drug or drugs of abuse that a patient has been using.

What then, is the clinician to do when faced with a patient who has been abstinent for a relatively short period of time (e.g., 10 days) and is complaining of depression? In such a case, since there is no clear guideline regarding the length of time necessary before a diagnosis can be made with absolute certainty, it is probably best to follow the patient longitudinally over time. As long as the patient's symptoms are improving as the result of abstinence alone, then it is probably not necessary to make an independent diagnosis of major depression and treat with antidepressants. If the patient's symptoms begin to worsen, however, then the likelihood of a coexisting disorder would increase. Moreover, it is highly unlikely that a worsening clinical picture after a period of improvement would be due to a withdrawal syndrome. Therefore, in such a case, the clinician can feel relatively confident concluding that another process is occurring concurrently.

COMPREHENSIVE TREATMENT APPROACHES

Despite the widespread prevalence of comorbid substance abuse and mood disorders, little research has been performed on the optimal treatment of this dually diagnosed population. The current clinical approach to treating such patients typically consists of a multidimensional treatment program with varying amounts of psychoeducation, psychotherapy, pharmacotherapy, and self-help groups.

For clinicians who treat this patient population, it is critical that treatment should focus specifically on both disorders. In treating a patient with alcoholism and major depression, for example, improvement in each disorder will clearly improve the prognosis of the other illness, but will not alleviate its symptoms completely. Thus, educating patients regarding the fact that they have two clinical diagnoses is an important early intervention. The clinician should discuss the nature of the two discrete disorders as well as reviewing the potential relationship between the two. Patients may react variably to this information; some may feel relieved, while others may experience this as an added burden. For example, certain alcoholics who have been stably sober but depressed may be accused by other members of Alcoholics Anonymous of wallowing in self-pity or not working the steps of the AA program properly. For these individuals, knowing that they have another treatable disorder may help relieve them from self-blame. Some patients with chronic psychiatric illness may, conversely, prefer the identity of being a substance abuser, although some may use this to deny their coexisting psychiatric disorder. Indeed, some patients may experience a phenomenon of "double denial," and question the validity of either diagnosis. For patients with two disorders, the process of acceptance may thus become either somewhat easier or far more difficult than for patients with only one diagnosis.

Psychotherapy

There is good research evidence that psychotherapy can be helpful in the treatment of patients with drug dependence and other psychopathology. For example, a study at the University of Pennsylvania (Woody et al., 1983) showed that opiate addicts in methadone maintenance treatment who had high levels of psychiatric severity fared better when treated with psychotherapy in addition to drug counseling than did similar patients who were treated with drug counseling alone.

One psychotherapeutic technique that can be useful in patients with coexisting substance use and mood disorders is to ask patients to present to their therapist a scenario by which they might relapse to either substance abuse or their mood disorder. Thus, for example, patients with bipolar disorder who are non-compliant with medications may be able to envision a relapse to hypomania, and a subsequent relapse to alcohol or drugs as the result of poor judgment. In this way, patients who may be motivated for the treatment of only one of two disorders (for example, a patient who knows he must stop drinking but is reluctant to take lithium, or a patient who is afraid of becoming depressed but thinks that "social drinking" is not problematic) may see the linkage between the two disorders.

Pharmacotherapy

Pharmacotherapy of patients with mood disorders and substance abuse is a subject that has generated a good deal of research interest. However, many of the studies that have been done on this subject, particularly studies of the pharmacotherapy of depression and alcoholism, have been flawed. The use of various methodologies to diagnose depression, failure to measure plasma antidepressant levels, and inconsistent treatment outcome measures have hindered many of these studies (Jaffe & Ciraulo, 1986). Nonetheless, recent research has shown some benefit in the use of antidepressants in alcoholics with coexisting major depression (Mason & Kocsis, 1991).

Several specific points must be borne in mind when treating depressed substance abusers with antidepressants. First, treatment with tricyclic antidepressants may lead to the so-called early tricyclic jitteriness syndrome, which may cause increased craving in stimulant abusers because of the similarity between tricyclic-induced jitteriness and stimulant-induced effects. Second, enhanced metabolism of tricyclic antidepressants may occur as the result of induction of hepatic enzymes by chronic heavy drinking. Therefore, higher than usual doses of certain antidepressants may be necessary when treating depressed patients with alcoholism; obtaining antidepressant blood levels may thus be important in treating these patients. Finally, the use of monoamine oxidase inhibitors must be considered cautiously in this population because of their frequent impulsive behavior, as well as the possibility that the use of stimulant drugs and/or certain alcoholic beverages may provoke hypertensive crises in patients taking these medications.

The treatment of patients with bipolar disorder and substance abuse can also be quite difficult. For example, although an earlier study suggested that lithium was beneficial in the treatment of cocaine abusers with bipolar disorder, more recent research (Nunes, McGrath, Wager & Quitkin, 1990) found that lithium had little efficacy in improving drug use in a group of cocaine abusers who had either cyclothymia or bipolar II disorder. Patients with bipolar disorder and substance abuse may have difficulty accepting both clinical conditions, and thus the need for pharmacologic treatment. Goodwin and Jamison (1990) have emphasized the importance of educating all patients with bipolar disorder, whether or not they have a coexisting substance use disorder, on a number of important aspects of drinking: a) that the combination of alcohol and lithium has an additive, often synergistic effect; b) that lithium may reduce the euphoria of drinking; c) that lithium may increase thirst or decrease alcohol's psychological effect, resulting in increased drinking; d) that alcohol can cause significant mood changes; e) that alcohol may alter sleep, which may aggravate a patient's mood disorder; f) that drinking alcohol may reduce compliance with medication treatment; g) that drinking may adversely affect prognosis; and h) that alcohol may have a deleterious effect on the efficacy of medication regimens. Finally, in selecting an anticonvulsant that may be used to supplement or replace lithium in the treatment of patients with bipolar disorder, there is evidence that the use of valproic acid may be preferable to carbamazepine in the treatment of opioid dependent patients receiving methadone maintenance treatment (Saxon, Whittaker, & Hawker, 1989). Since carbamazepine induces hepatic microsomal enzymes, this process may accelerate the metabolism of methadone, thus causing patients to experience opioid abstinence symptoms. Valproic acid is therefore generally the anticonvulsant of choice in this patient population.

Self-Help Groups

In addition to psychotherapeutic and pharmacologic treatment approaches, self-help groups are frequently utilized in the treatment of dually diagnosed patients. Although there has been some historical antagonism between mental health clinicians and self-help groups, this attitude of distrust has been gradually replaced with a sense of mutual respect for the unique qualities of each form of treatment. Nonetheless, some well meaning self-help group members will still challenge depressed patients who are taking medications and encourage them to stop "chewing their booze." Although AA literature such as "The AA Member-Medications and Other Drugs" clearly states that patients should follow their doctors' medication regimens, individuals in AA do not necessarily represent AA itself.

In recent years, some self-help groups (e.g., "Double Trouble") have formed specifically for patients with dual disorders. Other self-help groups such as the Manic Depressive and Depressive Association (MDDA) have been held for patients with mood disorders; these groups frequently talk about the adverse effects of alcohol and drug use on the course of their illness, and can be very helpful for these patients.

Several caveats should be borne in mind when treating patients with mood disorders and substance use disorders who are attending self-help groups. First, some patients may find self-help programs discouraging, because they feel alienated from others when they fail to experience the dramatic improvement in the quality of their lives that other group members describe accompanying their sobriety. Indeed, the persistence of depression, despite regular attendance and maintenance of sobriety, may lead to accusations of indulging in self-pity. These kinds of situations may make dually diagnosed patients feel misunderstood and may increase the likelihood of their dropping out of treatment. On the other hand, self-help group meetings can be very helpful to such patients, because of their structure, hopeful message, clarity of intent, and provision of group support.

Clinicians should facilitate the entry of their patients into self-help groups by periodically inquiring about their meeting schedule and their attendance. Early on, patients should be encouraged to attend a variety of meetings in order to help them select specific meetings in which they feel comfortable. Therapists should explore patients' behavior at meetings, including whether they speak or socialize with members. Patients should be encouraged to obtain a sponsor and may require some specific coaching as to how to do so. Asking about patients' attitudes towards and participation at self-help groups at regular intervals may help to solidify attendance. For example, a depressed shy patient who sits alone at meetings may benefit from attending meetings with a sponsor who is familiar with other group members. A patient who becomes bored, depressed, and restless at large open meetings may benefit from switching to meetings with smaller attendance. To intervene effectively, clinicians should gain familiarity with principles of self-help groups by attending open meetings and reading basic AA literature.

CONCLUSION

Patients with concurrent mood disorders and substance use disorders require flexible, comprehensive, and multidimensional treatment approaches that vary over time. Clinicians treating such patients need to be familiar with the course of each illness, the potential interactions between the two, and the specific relationship between the two illnesses in the individual patient. By focusing on both this overview and the particular characteristics of the specific patient, an effective treatment program can be designed and tailored to the individual.

REFERENCES

Gawin, F.H., & Kleber, H.D. (1986). Abstinence symptomatology and psychiatric diagnoses in cocaine abusers: Clinical observations. *Archives of General Psychiatry. 43*, 107–113.

Goodwin F.K., & Jamison K.R. (1990). Treatment of Alcohol and Drug Abuse in Manic-Depressive Patients. pp. 763–768. *Manic-Depressive Illness.* New York: Oxford University Press.

Jaffe, J.H., & Ciraulo, D.A. (1986). R.E. Meyer, (Ed). Alcoholism and depression, In *Psychopathology and Addictive Disorders.* pp. 293–320, New York: Guilford Press.

Khantzian, E.J. (1985). The self-medication hypothesis of addictive disorders: Focus on heroin and cocaine dependence. *American Journal of Psychiatry. 142*, 1259–1264.

Khantzian, E.J. (1989). Addiction: Self-destruction or self-repair? *Journal of Substance Abuse Treatment. 6*, 75.

Marzuk, P.M., & Mann, J.J. (1988). Suicide and substance abuse. *Psychiatric Annals. 18*, 639–645.

Mason, B.J., & Kocsis, J.H. (1991). Desipramine treatment of alcoholism. *Psychopharmacology Bulletin. 27*(2), 155–161.

Nunes, E.V., McGrath, P.J., Wager, S., & Quitkin, F.M. (1990). Lithium treatment for cocaine abusers with bipolar spectrum disorders. *American Journal of Psychiatry, 147*(5), 655–657.

Regier, D.A., Farmer, M.E., Rae, D.S., Locke, B.Z., Keith, S.J., Judd, L.L., & Goodwin, F.K. (1990). Comorbidity of mental disorders with alcohol and other drug abuse. Results from the Epidemiological Catchment Area (ECA) Study. *Journal of the American Medical Association. 264*, 2511–2518.

Rounsaville, B.J., Anton, S.F., Carroll, K., Budde, D., Prusoff, B.A., & Gawin, F. (1991). Psychiatric diagnoses of treatment-seeking cocaine abusers. *Archives of General Psychiatry. 48*, 43–51.

Rounsaville, B.J., & Kleber, H.D. (1984). Psychiatric disorders and the course of opiate addiction: Preliminary findings on predictive significance and diagnostic stability, in ed. S.M. Mirin, *Substance Abuse and Psychopathology*, Washington, DC: American Psychiatric Press, Inc., pp. 134–151.

Saxon, A.J., Whittaker, S., & Hawker, C.S. (1989). Valproic acid, unlike other anticonvulsants has no effect on methadone metabolism: Two cases. *Journal of Clinical Psychiatry. 50*(6), 228–229.

Schuckit, M.A. (1985). The clinical implications of primary diagnostic groups among alcoholics. *Archives of General Psychiatry. 42*, 1043–1049.

Schuckit, M.A. (1989). Suicidal behavior and substance abuse. *Drug Abuse and Alcoholism Newsletter. 18*, 8.

Weiss, R.D., Mirin, S.M., Griffin, M.L., & Michael, J.L. (1988). Psychopathology in cocaine abusers: Changing trends, *Journal of Nervous and Mental Disease. 176*, 719–725.

Weiss, R.D., Mirin, S.M., & Griffin, M.L. (1992-a). Methodological considerations in the diagnosis of coexisting psychiatric disorders in substance abusers. *British Journal of Addiction, 87*, 179–187.

Weiss, R.D., Griffin, M.L., & Mirin, S.M. (1992-b). Drug abuse as self-medication for depression: An empirical study. *American Journal of Drug and Alcohol Abuse. 18*(2), 121–129.

Woody, G.E., Luborsky, L., McLellan, A.T., O'Brien, C.P., Beck, A.T., Blaine, J., Herman, I., & Hole, A. (1983). Psychotherapy for opiate addicts. Does it help? *Archives of General Psychiatry. 40*, 639–645.

NOTES

Supported by Grant DA-0940 and Grant 1 U01 DA-07693 from the National Institute on Drug Abuse; and a grant from the Dr. Ralph and Marian C. Falk Medical Research Trust.

8

The Comorbidity of Substance Use and Mental Illness Among Adolescents

JEANNETTE L. JOHNSON, NICOLE E. POSNER and JON E. ROLF

INTRODUCTION

Adolescence is a time of developmental growth earmarked by an elaborate transition from childhood to young adulthood. During this time, rapid biological fluctuations of puberty bring with it an increasing array of accompanying psychological changes (Lerner & Foch, 1987). Physical appearances and body sizes transform. Biological and psychological functioning may undergo rapid and sometimes dramatic fluctuations. Even though many adolescents show impressive resiliency during this period, for some adolescents the inherent difficulty of this transition age, combined with other individual, family, and environmental factors leads to a pattern of high risk behavior. For these high risk youth, early adolescence becomes a period of extraordinary stress characterized by a variety of social, behavioral, and health problems. Some of these problems include the use of alcohol, tobacco, or illicit drugs; poor nutrition and exercise habits; early and unprotected sexual activity leading to unwanted pregnancies and sexually transmitted diseases including HIV/AIDS; delinquency; and violent, destructive, or suicidal behaviors.

There has been an increasing awareness that early problem behaviors, if left untreated, place youth at risk for enduring problems that last well into adulthood and consequently involve criminal and antisocial behaviors, chemical dependence, and mental illness (Rutter, Grahm, Chadick & Yale, 1976). As has been discussed in Chapter 2, epidemiologic studies provide some evidence that substance use predicts an increased risk of psychotic disorders (Tien & Anthony, 1990; Andersson, Allebect, Engstrom & Rydberg, 1987). These public health problems of high risk youth have been targeted for prevention and treatment programs. For example, in 1986, the enactment of Public Law 99-750, the "Anti-Drug Abuse Act", mandated that one of the priority target audiences would be high risk youth. In P.L. 99-750, a high risk youth is defined as an individual who has not attained the age of 21 years, who is at high risk of becoming, or who has become, a drug abuser or an alcohol abuser, and who (1) is identified as a child of a substance abuser; (2) is a victim of physical, sexual, or psychological abuse; (3) has dropped out of school; (4) has become pregnant; (5) is economically disadvantaged; (6) has committed a violent or delinquent act; (7) has experienced mental health problems; (8) has attempted suicide; or (9) is disabled by injuries.

The evidence for adolescent high risk behavior is startling, both in terms of its prevalence and consequence. Out of the 28 million US adolescents aged 10 to 17, Dryfoos (1987) estimated (based on 1984–1985 statistics) that: 5.7 million were behind in school, with 1.2 million two or more years behind, and 620,000 drop outs; 2.4 million used marijuana; 5.5 million drank alcohol and about half of these (2.4 million) were daily heavy drinkers; 3.1 million smoked cigarettes; 800,000 used multiple illicit drugs; 400,000 used cocaine; 4.8 million were sexually active; the estimated 1.8 million sexually active females resulted in 400,000 pregnancies, 177,000 births, and 176,000 abortions; 2 million adolescents were serious offenders; and 1.5 million adolescents were arrested.

There is converging evidence about these adolescent problems that suggests that many negative behavioral outcomes are interrelated (Bachman, O'Malley, & Johnston, 1980; Jessor & Jessor, 1977). Specifically, teens who are engaged in one type of problem behavior are often engaged in other problem behaviors (Elliott, Huizinga, & Ageton, 1985). This chapter examines the co-occurrence of two common problem behaviors of adolescence: *substance abuse* and *serious mental disorders*. These two areas are of increasing concern and appear to underlie or be associated with many other health compromising behaviors. We begin by examining the current prevalence data in each area. Next, we discuss current research examining the co-occurrence of problem behaviors with attention to the co-occurrence of substance abuse and mental disorders. Finally, we discuss promising treatment approaches that address the co-occurrence of substance abuse and mental disorders in adolescents.

Prevalence of Substance Use and Abuse in Adolescence

The large subgroup of adolescents in the U.S. population that abuses drugs cuts across social, ethnic, and geographic boundaries. Semlitz and Gold (1986) have examined the changing patterns of drug abuse among adolescents and young adults, and they conclude that there is no one prototypical adolescent drug abuser. It has been reported that youth from the U.S. have the highest rates of substance use of all industrialized nations (Irwin & Ryan, 1989). In general, and in spite of a recent decline in the use of some drugs (e.g., cocaine), experimentation and regular use of substances remains high among the general population of in-school U.S. adolescents, as shown by the annual High School Senior Class Surveys sponsored by the National Institute of Drug Abuse (Johnston, O'Malley & Bachman, 1992). The substances most frequently used in the Class of 1991 were: marijuana, inhalants, stimulants, hallucinogens, cocaine, and tranquilizers. In 1991, the lifetime prevalence (ever used) among high school seniors was 88 percent for alcohol, 36.7 percent for marijuana, 15.4 percent for stimulants, and 7.8 percent for cocaine. In this nation-wide survey of approximately 15,000 high school seniors (Class of 1991), 88% reported drinking alcohol during their lifetime; 38% first experienced drinking in the 6th–8th grades, and; 44% of high school seniors reported use of at least one illicit drug. Over a quarter of all seniors reported having used an illicit drug other than marijuana at some time.

Alcohol and tobacco are still the most widely abused substances among adolescents, but according to the 1992 NIDA survey, the prevalence rates have dropped each year since 1987. Nevertheless, more than two-thirds of 12 to 17 year olds used alcohol in the past year (from 1987), and about one-third of this group are current drinkers. Alcohol use continues to begin at younger and younger ages — the mean age of first use is 12.3 years, although some place that age as low as eight (Metropolitan Life, 1987).

Prevalence of Mental Disorders in Adolescence

Theories about the origins and consequences of psychopathology in all children are quite varied (Cowan, 1988; Johnson, Sher & Rolf, 1992). Nevertheless, despite the approximate 28 million adolescents in the United States, epidemiologic data on the prevalence of mental disorders during adolescence are limited. This general lack of research on mental health problems is alarming, given available information on rates of mental disorders during adolescence. Estimates suggest that approximately one out of every five adolescents have experienced or suffered from an emotional or behavioral problem (Costello, 1989; Kazdin, 1993; Zill & Schoenborn, 1990). Furthermore, the Office of Technology Assessment (1986) estimates that about twelve percent (7.5 million youth) of children under the age of 18 have a diagnosable mental disorder.

While depression is relatively rare in childhood, its incidence and prevalence increase during adolescence. The estimates of lifetime prevalence of depression among adolescents are startling. For example, by estimating the rate of depression from six adolescent clinical samples, Petersen, Compas, Brooks-Gunn, Stemmler, Ey and Grant, (1993) calculated it to be 42 percent. Adolescent suicide attempts, often associated with depression, peak at the ages of 15–19; 6–13 percent of adolescents have reported that they attempted suicide at least once in their lives (Shaffer, Vieland, Gorland, Rojas, Underwood & Busner, 1990).

Another way to quage mental disorders during adolescence is by examining the increasing incidence of adolescent admissions to psychiatric treatment. There has been a sharp rise in use of psychiatric treatment centers that are specifically designated for youth (Lerman, 1989). Since 1971, and especially since 1980, juvenile admissions to private hospitals have risen dramatically. Juvenile admissions to private psychiatric hospitals jumped at least 350 percent between 1980 and 1984. In 1980, about 81,532 juveniles were hospitalized for psychiatric treatment. Almost half of these admissions were for "preadult and other nonpsychotic" disorders that include adjustment reactions, childhood emotional disturbances, depression, conduct disorders, and a range of other problems (Jackson-Beeck, Schwartz & Rutherford, 1987). Additionally, the number of children in placement for emotional problems has risen dramatically over the past few years. Those in placement represent only a fraction of the 7.5 million American children believed to suffer from a mental health problem severe enough to require treatment (Select Committee on Children, Youth & Families, 1989).

Co-Occurring Problems

Studies of adult substance abusers have demonstrated the frequent co-occurrence of psychiatric and substance use disorders (Rounsaville, Weissman, Kleber & Wilber, 1982). Data from the Epidemiologic Catchment Area (ECA) studies, for example, show that over 25% of adults diagnosed with a psychiatric disorder are also diagnosed with a substance use disorder (Regier et al., 1990). Co-occurring substance use and mental disorders have been clinically recognized in adolescents, but we know less about the prevalence of this co-occurrence than we do in adults (Belfer, 1993). Little is known about the specific co-occurrence of mental disorders and substance abuse in the adolescent population, the developmental progress into multiproblem patterns, and whether or not the problems are related to one another, independent, or different manifestations of a common syndrome (Elliott, Huizinga, & Menard, 1988). Each area of problem behaviors has generated its own separate research literature based on the history and tradition of the field; thus, we have separate information for adolescent pregnancy, juvenile delinquency, substance abuse, runaways, academic failures, and psychopathology. In view of recent findings, these divisions appear to be artificial (Elliott et al., 1985; Jessor & Jessor, 1977). For example, in a community sample of 11 year olds diagnosed with a psychiatric disorder, almost 55% had more than one diagnosis (Andersen, Williams, McGee & Silva, 1987).

Co-occurring adolescent problems have been discussed at great length by Jessor and Jessor (1977) who suggest the existence of a syndrome of adolescent problem behaviors that consists of drinking, problem drinking, marijuana use, delinquency, and early sexual intercourse. Their longitudinal data on senior high school and college students showed that problem behaviors correlated positively with each other and correlated negatively with conventional behaviors (e.g., church attendance). Hundleby (1987) replicated these findings in a sample of 1,048 14 year olds and reported that sexual behavior, delinquency, and maladaptive social behavior were major correlates of marijuana, alcohol, and tobacco use. Other research shows that problem behaviors frequently co-occur during adolescence that includes alcohol use, cigarette smoking, marijuana use, use of other illicit drugs, delinquent behavior, and precocious sexual intercourse (Bachman et al., 1980; Elliott et al., 1985).

SUBSTANCE ABUSE AND MENTAL ILLNESS

Little is known about the specific relationship between substance abuse and mental illness in adolescence. Two reasons are partially responsible for our lack of information. First, recognition of the co-occurrence of substance abuse and mental illness in adolescents is only recent (Belfer, 1993). Second, the major impediment to understanding the co-occurrence is the absence of an appropriate and useful nosology for diagnosing adolescent substance use and abuse, as well as mental illness (Belfer, 1993; Halikas, Lyttle, Morse & Hoffman, 1984).

While there is substantial clinical evidence of substance use disorders in adolescents who are also diagnosed with a mental illness, there is little information on the prevalence of this co-occurrence and few systematic studies of this relationship (Belfer, 1993; Bukstein, Brent & Kaminer, 1989). Studying adolescent substance abuse shows that it is a pervasive problem during adolescence, and evidence of the co-occurrence of substance abuse with almost every type of diagnosable mental illness proliferates (Kaminer, 1991). This makes it difficult to distinguish the specificity of the relationships between substance abuse and particular diagnoses of mental illness. For example, among recently detoxified adolescent inpatient substance abusers, DeMilio (1989) reported that the most prevalent psychiatric diagnoses were: conduct disorder (42%), major depression (35%), and a combination of attention deficit, hyperactivity, or impulsive disorder (21%). Similarly, in a review of adolescent psychiatric diagnosis among emergency room admissions, patients with secondary psychiatric diagnosis to alcoholism were classified with either depression or conduct disorder (Reichler, Clement, & Dunner, 1983). In 1988, 38 percent of adolescent psychiatric admissions to city hospitals were crack-related, up from 18 percent in 1987 (Plaut & Kelly, 1989). However, due to the complexities involved with retrospective reporting of behaviors, problems with adolescent diagnostic procedures, and differences in research methodologies, many studies of adolescent comorbidity are inconsistent. Some studies show weak positive associations between substance abuse and mental health problems (McLaughlin, Bauer, Burside & Pokorny, 1985; Paton, Kessler, & Kandel, 1977). The research that has examined the relationship between substance abuse and psychiatric diagnosis among adolescents has examined such things as hyperactivity, conduct problems, juvenile delinquency, and depression. The association between hyperactivity and substance abuse is unclear (Milin, Halikas, Meller & Morse, 1991). Some studies report no association (Weiss & Hectman, 1986) while others find significant relationships (Gittelman, Mannuzza, Shenker & Bonagura, 1985). Similarly, the relationship between substance abuse and conduct problems (Bukstein et al., 1989; Stewart, Deblois & Cumming, 1980) is ambiguous surprising in view of the findings suggesting that substance abuse and antisocial personality are strongly associated (Lewis, Rice & Helzer, 1983; Shuckit, 1982). This notion is confirmed by the conspicuous relationship between juvenile delinquency and drug use (Chein, Gerard, Lee & Rosenfeld, 1964; Elliot & Ageton, 1976; Johnston, O'Malley & Eveland, 1978). In one study (Milin et al., 1991), 81% of juvenile offenders met a diagnosis of substance abuse; approximately three-fourths of this substance abusing group showed evidence of psychopathology.

Depression is frequently noted in substance abusing adolescents both in the general population and in psychiatric treatment (Belfer, 1993). Kashani, Keller, Solomon, Reid and Mazzola (1985) showed that double depression (dysthymic disorder with superimposed major depression) that lasted at least a year could be detected in 16% of the adolescent substance abusers frequenting a youth drop-in counseling center. Deykin, Levy and Wells (1987) showed that both alcohol and other drug abuse were associated with major depressive disorder in a sample of 424 older adolescents (16 to 19 years old). The prevalence of major depressive disorder in this sample was 6.8 percent; alcohol abuse was 8.2 percent and substance abuse was 9.4 percent. These findings were uniquely related to the type of substance abused. Alcohol abuse was associated with major depression, but drug (other than alcohol) abuse was related to other psychiatric diagnoses.

One study by Elliot and colleagues (1988) showed that the highest prevalence of alcohol, marijuana, polydrug, and problem substance use was found among adolescents with both serious delinquency and emotional problems. In a community sample of adolescent delinquency, substance abuse, and mental illness, they concluded that adolescents tended to have higher prevalence rates for problem substance abuse and mental health service utilization if they also had emotional problems. Moreover, there was a curvilinear relationship between age and delinquency; delinquency peaked in mid-adolescence. Age and drug use were positively related and leveled off or reversed in young adulthood. They found no significant relationships between mental health problems and age.

TREATMENT FOR CO-OCCURRING MENTAL ILLNESS AND SUBSTANCE ABUSE IN ADOLESCENTS

The combined effects of mental illness and substance abuse in adolescents have devastating consequences. These youth have severe and complex problems which, if left untreated, may continue long into adulthood. The Center for Substance Abuse Treatment (CSAT, 1991) recently identified some promising treatment approaches for these adolescents that range from short-term school-based interventions to long-term residential therapeutic communities. The most effective of these programs have multiple treatment approaches that integrate legal, health, recreational, and educational services; some programs use therapeutic foster parents. Although the programs differ in many ways, efficacious programs uphold certain similarities such as group therapy (either peer counseling or self-help groups), family involvement, and the recognition that recovery is a process.

The CSAT (1991) report recommends programs for dually diagnosed adolescents that are intensive and long-term; these types of programs allow behavioral changes to become internalized. Therapeutic approaches should treat the adolescent as a whole person through comprehensive, integrated, and accessible services. A wide range of services and activities (special and vocational education, birth control services, or recreational activities) enable adolescents to explore alternative lifestyles, engage in constructive relationships, and plan for independent, drug-free living. The length of treatment should vary according to the severity of adolescent abuse problems, mental health, and home and school environment. Aftercare is an essential component to any successful adolescent treatment program because even though some adolescents do well in treatment, many relapse upon returning to the original environment. Strong transition and aftercare components can reduce the chance of relapse and help to ensure continuity of treatment goals. Finally, they recommend that culturally sensitive HIV/AIDS education should be provided throughout the program that is coupled with strong, open-ended educational efforts focusing on the dynamics of relationships and the responsibilities associated with relationships.

The CSAT (1991) report describes two basic categories of treatment programs for dually diagnosed adolescents. The first category, clinic and day treatment programs, involve five different types of strategies. **School-based strategies** (e.g., Matrix Community Services in Tucson, Arizona) provide drug treatment and interventions in schools that consist of alcohol and drug education, peer counseling, and alternative activities that are designed to effect schoolwide attitude changes. **Comprehensive broad services** provide 'one-stop' comprehensive services to adolescents in a youth center environment. This approach emphasizes serving the whole person with a wide range of programs (including legal, social work, health, educational, and mental health) that integrates substance abuse and mental health services into an overall treatment plan. **Targeted subpopulation** approaches provide counseling services to specific subpopulations of adolescents, such as those who have been sexually abused and are substance abusers. Receiving treatment for a specific problem concurrently with treatment for the addiction helps the client to remain drug and alcohol free during treatment. **Clinic and partial day treatment** centers offer different levels of individualized treatment ranging from a 10-week drug education outpatient program to partial day treatment for only three days a week. The treatment plan can be continually altered, depending on the individual's needs and treatment progress. **Culturally specific outpatient treatment** (such as the Mainstream Youth Program in Portland, Oregon) provides outpatient substance abuse treatment, education, and prevention programming for African-American youth. This type of treatment uses community outreach and culturally specific approaches to address the special needs of inner-city adolescents.

The second category of treatment services, residential programs, also include several different strategies. **Combined day and residential treatment** (e.g., Threshold for Change in Novato, California), provides comprehensive treatment programming with a range of services for local communities that includes day treatment, residential care, and case management. **Dual-diagnosis** (e.g., West Prep Adolescent Day Treatment Program in Valhalla, New York) programs are designed to meet the needs of the formally dually diagnosed adolescent through a combination of mental health day treatment with substance abuse counseling, education, occasional training, and recreation in a year-long day treatment program. **Short-term inpatient** programs generally serve adolescents on an inpatient partial hospitalization unit. Typically, after discharge, intensive day treatment and outpatient care are provided for a year or longer.

Day treatment and therapeutic foster care, such as that offered at the Morrison Center in Portland, Oregon, typically serves drug abusing criminally involved adolescents. **Therapeutic Community and aftercare**, such as that provided by Amity, Inc., in Tucson, Arizona, is a typical therapeutic community that provides substance abuse services to adolescents. **Long-term residential and transitional apartments** (i.e., Pahl House of Troy, New York) are long-term residential programs that provide a transitional residences for adolescents. Some adolescents may spend up to several years in transitional apartments. **State level initiatives** (i.e., the Alaska Youth Initiative in Juno, Alaska) coordinate services for difficult-to-serve adolescents using various interventions that are based on flexible, personalized, and local treatment principles.

THE COMPLEX RELATIONSHIP BETWEEN SUBSTANCE ABUSE AND MENTAL ILLNESS IN ADOLESCENCE: A RESEARCH, PREVENTION, AND TREATMENT PUZZLE

Substance abuse underlies many serious problems of adolescence, and perhaps it is just one problem in a long list of potential adolescent problems. For example, the leading cause of death for adolescents is injury, either through accidents, car crashes, homicide, or suicide. In 1986, 80% of the deaths among adolescents were from accidents, homicides, and suicides; an increase of 51% from 1950 (Irwin & Ryan, 1989). Many of these injuries and deaths are associated with alcohol or other drug abuse, which is highly pervasive among the adolescent population as a whole. In the U.S., the high rate of school dropout, an alarming precursor to unemployability and poverty, is another example of the potential underlying effects of substance abuse. In some inner cities and rural areas, the dropout rate is over 50 percent (Sherman, 1987). Most national surveys conclude that the overall dropout rate is between 13 and 18 percent, with higher rates for males than females, and higher rates for all minorities except Asians (Sherman, 1987).

The complex relationship between substance abuse and mental illness in adolescence is most likely consists of multiple etiologies that take multiple paths of expression (Newcomb & Bentler, 1989). A simple univariate relationship between substance abuse and mental illness is unlikely to exist (Greenbaum, Prange, Friedman, & Silver, 1991). Separating the normal developmental fluctuations of adolescent behavior from abnormal behavioral patterns is illusive, at best; understanding how children develop substance abuse or psychopathology, and how this co-occurs, requires a simultaneous understanding of a broad array of developmental factors. We need to understand how biological and psychological processes combine with one another and with the socio-cultural environment to affect the day to day and year to year progression of the child's behavior.

Many methodological problems have slowed the advance of research. Because most studies are univariate, they preclude an integration of biological, psychological, and social perspectives. Small sample sizes employed in the majority of studies are a major problem because these designs suffer from limited statistical power. Also, there are potential problems associated with the selection of control groups. Matching on sociodemographic variables does not solve the potential problems inherent in comparing children whose parents are in treatment with children whose parents are not in treatment. At present, the methodological limitations in the existing research limit the types of generalizations we can make.

Future research on the relationship between substance abuse and psychopathology in adolescence needs to be attentive to the numerous issues raised by both traditional developmental research and psychopathological research on children. Because children change at varying degrees and rates, what may be normal for some children at one age is not normal for other children at the same age, depending on individual rates of development and environmental context. Thus, it is difficult to determine the boundaries of normal age-appropriate behavior. Added to this difficulty is the task of understanding childhood behavioral deviation and its relationship to adulthood deviation. What is needed are longitudinal studies of larger samples to make possible comparisons to normative variations in development.

REFERENCES

Andersen, J.C., Williams, S., McGee, R., & Silva, P.A. (1987). DSM III disorders in preadolescent children: Prevalence in a large sample from the general population. *Archives of General Psychiatry.* 44, 69–76,

Andersson, S., Allebeck, P., Engstrom, A., & Rydberg, V., (1987). Cannabis and schizophrenia; A longitudinal study of Swedish conscripts. *Lancet.* December 26, 1483–1486.

Anti-Drug Abuse Act, Public Law #99-750 (1986).

Bachman, J. G., O'Malley P. M., & Johnston, L. D. (1980). *Correlates of drug use: Part 1. Selected measures of background, recent experiences, and lifestyle orientations* (Monitoring the Future, Occasional Paper No. 8). Ann Arbor, MI: Institute for Social research.

Belfer, M. L. (1993). Substance abuse with psychiatric illness in children and adolescents: Definitions and terminology. *American Journal of Orthopsychiatry, 63*(1), 70–79.

Bukstein, O. G., Brent, D. A., & Kaminer, Y. (1989). Comorbidity of substance abuse and other psychiatric disorders in adolescents. *American Journal of Psychiatry, 146*(9), 1131–1141.

Center for Substance Abuse Treatment (1991). Approaches in the Treatment of Adolescents with Emotional and Substance Abuse Problems. Technical Assistance Publication Series Number 1, DHHS Publication No. (SMA) 93–1744.

Chein, I., Gerard, D. L., Lee, R. S., & Rosenfeld, E. (1964). *The road to H: narcotics, delinquency, and social policy.* New York: Basic Books.

Costello, E. J. (1989). Developments in child psychiatric epidemiology. *Journal of the American Academy of Child and Adolescent Psychiatry, 28,* 836–841.

Cowan, P.A. (1988). Developmental psychopathology: A nine-cell map of the territory. In: Nannis, E.D., Cowan, P.A., eds. *Developmental Psychopathology and Its Treatment.* San Francisco: Jossey Bass, 1988. pp. 5–30.

DeMilio, L. (1989). Psychiatric syndromes in adolescent substance abusers. *American Journal of Psychiatry, 146*(9), 1212–1214.

Deykin, E. Y., Levy, J. C., & Wells, V. (1987). Adolescent depression, alcohol and drug abuse. *American Journal of Public Health, 77*(2), 178–182.

Dryfoos, J. (1987). *Youth at risk: One in four jeopardy.* Manuscript submitted for publication.

Elliott, D. S., & Ageton, A.R. (1976). The relationship between drug use and crime in adolescents. In: *Research Triangle Institute, appendix to drug use and crime: Report of the panel on drug use and criminal behavior.* Springfield, VA: National Technical Information Service, pp 297–322.

Elliott, D. S., Huizinga, D., & Ageton, A.R. (1985). *Explaining delinquency and drug use.* Beverly Hills, CA: Sage.

Elliott, D. S., Huizinga, D., & Menard, S. (1988). *Multiple problem youth: Delinquency, substance use, and mental health problems.* New York: Springer-Verlag.

Gittleman, R., Mannuzza, S., Shenker, R., & Bonagura, N. (1985). Hyperactive boys almost grown up, I: psychiatric status. *Archives of General Psychiatry, 42,* 937–947.

Greenbaum, P. E., Prange, M. E., Friedman, R. M., & Silver, S. E. (1991). Substance abuse prevalence and comorbidity with other psychiatric disorders among adolescents with severe emotional disturbances. *Journal of Acad. Child Adolesc. Psychiatry, 30*(4),42–56.

Halikas, J. A., Lyttle, M. D., Morse, C. L., & Hoffmann, R. G. (1984). Proposed criteria for the diagnosis of alcohol abuse in adolescents. *Comprehensive Psychiatry, 25*(6), 581–585.

Hamburg, D. A., & Takanishi, R. (1989). Preparing for life: The critical transition of adolescence. *American Psychologist, 44*(5), 825–842.

Irwin, C. E., & Ryan, S. A. (1989). Problem behavior of adolescents. *Pediatrics in Review, 10*(8), 235–246.

Jackson-Beeck, M., Schwartz, I. M., & Rutherford, A. (1987). Trends and issues in juvenile confinement for psychiatric ad chemical dependency treatment. *International Journal of Law and Psychiatry, 10,* 153–156.

Jessor, R., & Jessor, S. L. (1977). *Problem behavior and psychosocial development: A longitudinal study of youth.* New York: Academic Press.

Johnson, J.L., Sher, K.J., & Rolf, J.E. (1992). Models of vulnerability to psychopathology in children of alcoholics: An overview. *Alcohol Health and Research World, 15*(1), 32–42.

Johnston, L. D., O'Malley, P. M., & Bachman, J. G. (1992). *Drug use, drinking, and smoking: National survey results from high school, college, and young adult populations, 1975–1991.* Ann Arbor, MI: University of Michigan/Institute for Social Research (for NIDA).

Johnston, L. D., O'Malley, P. M., & Eveland, L. K. (1978). Drugs and delinquency: a search for causal connections. In D. B. Kandel(Ed.) *Longitudinal research on drug use: Empirical findings and methodological issues.* Washington DC: Hemisphere-John Wiley.

Kaminer, Y. (1991). The magnitude of concurrent psychiatric disorders in hospitalized substance abusing adolescents. *Child Psychiatry and Human Development, 22*(2), 89–95.

Kashani, J. H., Keller, M. B., Solomon, N., Reid, J. C., & Mazzola, D. (1985). Double depression in adolescent substance users. *Journal of Affective Disorders, 8,* 153–157.

Kazdin, A. E. (1993). Adolescent Mental Health Prevention and Treatment Programs. *American Psychologist, 48*(2), 127–141.

Lerman, P. (March 1989). Counting youth in trouble living away from home: Recent trends and counting problems. Center for the Study of Youth and Policy, Rutgers University. Unpublished Paper.

Lerner, R. M., & Foch, T. T. (1987). *Biological-psychosocial interactions in early adolescence.* Hillsdale, NJ: Lawrence Erlbaum Associates, Publishers.

Lewis, C. E., Rice, J., & Helzer, J. E., (1983). Diagnostic interactions: alcoholism and antisocial personality. *Journal Nerv. Met. Dis., 171,* 105–113.

McLaughlin, R. J., Baer, P. E., Burside, M. A., & Pokorny, A. D. (1985). Psychosocial correlates of alcohol use at two age levels during adolescence. *Journal of Studies on Alcohol, 46,* 212–218.

Metropolitan Life. (1987). Alcohol use among children and adolescents. *Statistical Bulletin, 68*(4).

Milin, R., Halikas, J. A., Meller, J. E., & Morse, C. (1991). Psychopathology among substance abusing juvenile offenders. *Journal of the American Academy of Child Adolescent Psychiatry. 30*(4), 569–574.

Newcomb, M.D., & Bentler, P.M. (1989). Substance use and abuse among children and teenagers. *American Psychologist, 44*(2), 242–248.

Office of Technology Assessment. (1986). Publication No. OTA-BP-H-33. U.S. Government Printing Office, Washington DC.

Paton, S. M., Kessler, R., & Kandel, D. B. (1977). Depressive mood and adolescent illicit drug use: A longitudinal study. *Journal of Genetic Psychology, 131,* 267–289.

Peterson, A. C., Compas, B. E., Brooks-Gunn, J., Stemmler, M., Ey, S., & Grant, K. E. (1993). Depression in adolescence. *American Psychologist, 48,* 155–168.

Plaut, J., & Kelley, T. (1989). *Childwatch: Children and Drugs,* New York: Interface.

Regier D. A., Farmer, M. E., Rae, D. S., Locke, D. Z., Keith, S. J., Judd, L. L., & Goodwin, F. K. (1990). Comorbidity of mental disorders and other drug abuse: Results from the epidemiologic catchment (ECA) study. *Journal of the Ameriacn Medical Association, 264*(19), 2511–2518.

Riechler, B. D., Clement, J. L., & Dunner, D. L. (1983). Chart Review of Alcohol Problems in Adolescent Psychiatric Patients in an Emergency Room. *Journal of Clinical Psychiatry, 44*(9), 338–339.

Rounsaville, B. J., Weissman, M. M., Kleber, H., & Wilber, C. (1982). Heterogeneity of psychiatric diagnosis in treated opiate addicts. *Archives of General Psychiatry, 39*, 161–166.

Rutter, M., Graham, P., Chadwick, O., & Yule, W. (1976). Adolescent turmoil: Fact or fiction? *Journal of Child Psychology and Psychiatry, 17*, 35–56.

Select Committee on Children, Youth, and Families (1989). A report with additional views of the Select Committee on Children, Youth, and Families, One Hundred First Congress. U.S. Children and Their Families: Current Conditions and Recent Trends, 1989. USGPO, #21–956.

Semlitz, L., & Gold, M. S. (1986). Adolescent drug abuse diagnosis, treatment, and prevention. *Psychiatric Clinics of North America, 9*(3), 455–473.

Shaffer, D., Vieland, V., Garland, A., Rojas, M., Underwood, M., & Busner, C. (1990). Adolescent suicide attempters: Response to suicide prevention programs. *Journal of the American Medical Association. 264*, 3151–3155.

Sherman, J. D. (1987). *Dropping out of school volume I: Causes and consequences for male and female youth.* Pelavin Associates, Inc., for the U.S. Department of Education.

Shuckit, M. A. (1982). A study of young men with alcoholic close relatives. *American Journal of Psychiatry, 139*, 791–794.

Stewart, M. A., Deblois, C. S., & Cummings, C. (1980). Psychiatric disorder in the parents of hyperactive boys and those with conduct problems. *Journal Child Psychol. Psychiatry, 21*, 283–292.

Tien, A.Y., & Anthony, J.C. (1990). Epidemiological analysis of alcohol and drug use as risk factors for psychotic experiences. *Journal of Nervous and Mental Disease, 178*, 473–480.

Weiss, G., & Hechtman, L. T. (1986). *Hyperactive children grown up.* New York: Guilford.

Zill, N., & Schoenborn, C. A. (1990, November). *Developmental, learning, and emotional problems: Health of our nation's children, United States 1988* (No. 190) Washington, DC: National Center for Health Statistics.

9

Dual Diagnosis in the Elderly

STEPHEN BARTELS and JOSEPH LIBERTO

INTRODUCTION

The high prevalence of comorbid psychiatric and substance use disorders is well-documented among younger age groups. However, little is known about elderly individuals with dual disorders. Demographic data show that those over age 65 are the fastest growing segment of the population, with estimates that this group will increase from 12% of the population currently, to over 21% by the year 2030 (Spencer, 1989). These future trends suggest the need for increased attention to the problem of alcohol and other drug abuse in the elderly.

There is little research pertaining to dual diagnosis in the elderly. This chapter highlights the small amount of available data on dual diagnosis in the elderly. For the purpose of discussion, the term "dual diagnosis" will be applied to substance use disorders and mental illness (excluding comorbid neurological conditions, dementia, or delirium) in keeping with the topical focus of other chapters in this book. Following this overview, the authors suggest factors to be considered in developing diagnostic and treatment guidelines for

139

this group of patients. Finally, clinical questions are considered that may help to shape the future research directions.

Epidemiology

Epidemiological data relevant to psychiatric and substance use comorbidity in the elderly come from several different perspectives. Sources include samples with primary psychiatric diagnoses, samples with primary substance abuse diagnoses, community population samples, and longitudinal outcome studies.

Psychiatric Samples

Research on elderly persons with mental illness have neglected comorbid substance use disorders, with the exception of several key studies. In general, these reports share the common finding of an association between affective disorders and alcohol abuse in elderly people treated in institution-based (residential or hospital) settings. For example, a review of the medical records of 128 patients age 55 and older in an intensive residential psychiatric treatment program found that 21% of the sample had comorbid psychiatric and substance use disorders, including 42% of patients with a personality disorder, 20% of patients with bipolar disorder, 16% of patients with major depression, and 13% of patients with a primary diagnosis of schizophrenia. Overall, the most frequent configuration of co-morbid disorders involved the three diagnoses of major depression, alcoholism and personality disorder (Speer & Bates, 1992).

Similarly, a study of 90 elderly psychiatric inpatients (age 65 or older) admitted primarily for treatment of depression or organic mental disorder, reported substantial comorbidity with 21% of patients meeting criteria for dependence on alcohol or drugs. Unfortunately, exact frequencies of specific psychiatric disorders were not reported. In this study, benzodiazepine dependence was the most common substance use disorder, occurring in 18% (N=16) of the total sample, including 10 patients who had drug dependence that was not recognized by the treating clinicians (Whitcup & Miller, 1987). Finally, a prospective study of 58 psychiatric inpatients over age 55 with depression found that a past history of alcoholism was a major risk factor for chronicity of depression assessed at four-year follow-up (Cook, Winokur, Garvey & Beach, 1991).

Substance Abuse Samples

Few data exist on the prevalence of major psychiatric illness among elderly individuals with primary substance abuse diagnoses. A relevant study by Finlayson, Hurt, Lavis and Morse, (1988) retrospectively reviewed the medical records of 216 subjects, age 65 and older, admitted to a 28-day alcohol dependence rehabilitation treatment program. The authors found that 44% of the sample had a comorbid organic brain syndrome diagnosis (i.e. dementia, delirium, amnestic syndrome and atypical organic brain syndrome), 12% had comorbid affective disorders (major depression being the most prevalent), 3% had a personality disorder, and less than 1% had a comorbid anxiety disorder. The high prevalence of organicity found in this study is consistent with neuropsychological studies of individuals with long-term, chronic alcohol use disorders who are more likely to exhibit cognitive deficits in the areas of visuospatial, memory, and perceptual motor function (Tarter & Ryan, 1983). A study of 281 homeless older men similarly found that alcoholism was associated with depression, yet found no association with organic mental disorder or psychosis and past psychiatric hospitalization (Cohen, Teresi & Holmes, 1988). Finally, Krystal and colleagues (1992) reported on the effects of age and alcoholism on the prevalence of panic disorder in the Epidemiologic Catchment Area (ECA) study. Among older adults, the six month prevalence rates of comorbid alcohol use disorder and panic disorder was 7.6% for women age 55 to 64, but there was no comorbid panic disorder for men in the same age group and for men and women age 65 and older.

Community Samples

ECA data reports of prevalence rates of current alcohol use disorders among those age of 65 or over (irrespective of comorbid psychiatric illness) range from 1.9 to 4.6% for men, and 0.1% to 0.7% for women (Myers et al., 1984). Over 10% of the elderly seeking medical treatment have alcohol use disorders (Beresford, Blow, Bower, Adams & Hall, 1988), and rates are even higher among V.A. and inner city public hospitals where the prevalence is over 20% (Curtis, Geller, Stokes, Levine & Moore, 1989). ECA studies of non-prescription drug abuse in the community found no evidence of drug abuse in adults age 65 or older at two of the three ECA sites, and a prevalence of 0.2% at the third. Lifetime prevalence was only 0.1% for these subjects at the three sites (Robins, Helzer & Przybeck, 1988). Though non-prescription drug abuse is rare in the elderly, it is estimated that 25% of older adults (over age 55) use psychoactive drugs with the associated risk of prescribed drug dependence and abuse (Beardsley, Gordocki, Larson & Hidalgo, 1988). Furthermore, higher lifetime prevalence rates of alcohol use disorders and drug abuse in younger individuals in the population suggest that cohort differences in drinking and drug use may result in higher rates of substance use disorders in future generations of the elderly (Blazer, 1989).

The few available studies of comorbid mental illness and substance abuse in elderly community samples suggest an association between affective disorders and alcohol abuse, though the data are inconclusive. For example, in a community survey of 997 elderly people over age 64, a history of alcohol abuse was uncommon (occurring in only 4.5% of the sample), yet almost half of this subgroup (2% of the total sample) reported comorbid depression or dysphoria (Blazer & Williams, 1980). A somewhat higher prevalence comorbidity was found in a select, community sample of 1668 elderly (over age 60) who were identified as high-risk, multiply impaired, and requiring in-home services of a specialized multidisciplinary outreach team (Jinks & Raschko, 1990). This chart review study found that 9.6% of the sample had alcohol abuse, and almost two-thirds of the alcohol abusing subgroup (6% of the the total sample) had comorbid psychiatric illness including depression (2.7%), bipolar disorder (0.7%), dementia (1.9%), schizophrenia (0.5%), and anxiety disorder (0.2%). This study also found that 5% of the total sample had a prescription drug abuse diagnosis (most frequently diazepam and codeine), yet comorbid psychiatric illness was not reported. Overall, these two studies suggest that alcohol abuse affects a small percentage of community-residing elderly, yet within this subgroup, comorbid psychiatric disorders are common. In contrast to these studies, no association was found between depression scores and alcohol consumption in a study of 1617 community-residing elderly (age 65 or older), except for women with moderate consumption (once or twice a week) who had significantly lower rates of depressive symptoms compared to women who never drank (Palinkas, Wingard & Barrett-Conner, 1990).

Longitudinal Studies

Longitudinal studies are essential to understanding the impact of aging. Long-term studies of the natural history of alcoholism show that roughly 2–3% become abstinent each year, with 10 to 15 years of severe alcohol abuse often preceding stable abstinence (Vaillant, 1983). Long-term outcome studies on comorbid substance abuse and severe mental illness are lacking (Turner & Tsuang, 1990). Available retrospective studies are limited to comparisons between schizophrenic patients who have recovered from prior substance use disorders and those without a lifetime history of substance abuse, showing few differences in outcomes (Zisook, Heaton, Mornaville, Kuck, Jernigan & Braff, 1992; Bartels, Drake & Wallach, 1995).

Longitudinal prospective data are few and include studies of samples primarily with affective disorders, and samples primarily with schizophrenia or schizoaffective disorder. Loosen, Dew and Prange (1990) reported poor outcomes in middle-aged men with a history of co-morbid depression and alcoholism (mean age = 50) followed over two years after achieving stable abstinence. Hasin, Endicott and Keller (1991) followed the course of alcohol problems in a sample of patients with affective syndromes over 5 years (two-thirds < age 40) and found that alcohol dependence, previous chronicity of alcohol problems, and a diagnosis of schizoaffective disorder predicted poor outcome. The cumulative probability of remission for at least 6 months over the five years of follow-up was .90, yet among those who remitted, the cumulative probability of subsequent relapse was .50. Finally, a recently completed seven-year follow-up study of a sample of patients primarily diagnosed with schizophrenia and schizoaffective disorder (mean age = 47 at follow-up) found relatively little change in the overall rate of substance use disorder from baseline to follow-up (31% vs. 27%), and poor outcomes among severely mentally ill substance abusers at follow-up including increased psychiatric symptoms, poor psychosocial function and greater treatment noncompliance. (Bartels, Drake & Wallach, 1993).

CLINICAL CONSIDERATIONS

Physiological Factors, Aging, and Dual Diagnosis

Physiological changes associated with aging result in a progressive decrease in capacity to handle alcohol and other drugs with a corresponding increased sensitivity to adverse effects. Potential interactions of prescribed medications coupled with declining ability to metabolize alcohol or other drugs make the elderly highly vulnerable to medical complications and toxicity. Physiological changes associated with aging include reduced hepatic metabolism and renal clearance causing substances to stay in the body for longer periods; reduced lean body mass and plasma albumin coupled with an increase in the ratio of water compartment to total body mass resulting in increased concentrations of drugs in the blood; and increased neuroreceptor sensitivity to psychotropic agents resulting in heightened therapeutic and toxic response to alcohol and other drugs (Abernathy, 1992).

The dually diagnosed elderly patient may be particularly prone to adverse effects of drugs or alcohol. In addition to the increased biological sensitivity to substances due to age described above, the presence of severe mental illness may create an additional biological vulnerability. Even small amounts of psychoactive substances may have adverse effects for individuals with schizophrenia and other brain disorders (Drake, Osher & Wallach, 1989). Consequently, the metabolic and physiological changes of aging, combined with increased sensitivity to alcohol or other drugs associated with severe mental illness, may result in a compounded risk for adverse effects from small amounts of substances.

Assessment

Alcohol and other substance use disorders are under-recognized in older persons (Curtis et al., 1989; Zimberg, 1987). Several factors contribute to failures in diagnosis. First, diagnostic criteria appropriate to younger populations do not always apply to the older population. For example, the ability to develop tolerance and dependence decreases with older age, making these signs poor markers for alcohol and other substance use disorders (Miller, 1991). Similarly, DSM-III-R criteria stress consequences of alcohol and drug use that are less useful indicators in the elderly. Elderly individuals are more likely to live alone, to be unemployed, and less likely to drive and experience legal problems related to drug or alcohol abuse (Miller, 1991). Second, signs of alcohol or drug abuse may be misinterpreted as a product of "normal aging" or medical illness, including affective changes, social isolation, and cognitive impairment (Zimberg, 1987). Finally, countertransference issues, coupled with rationalization of not wanting to take away an older persons' "few remaining pleasures," may set the stage for observer denial and enabling activity by relatives, friends and clinicians.

The same factors contributing to failures in detection of alcohol or substance use disorders in the elderly are shared by individuals with severe mental illness, who are also more likely to be single, isolated, unemployed, often do not drive cars, and are likely to have symptoms of substance abuse misinterpreted as an exacerbation of their underlying mental disorder. Similar countertransference issues may occur. As substance abuse is typically under-diagnosed in persons with severe mental illness (Ananth, Vandewater, Kamal, Brodsky, Gamal & Miller, 1989) and in elderly populations (Zimberg, 1987), it is likely that non-detection is common in patients who are both elderly and dually diagnosed.

Depression and anxiety are the most common psychiatric symptoms resulting from alcohol, sedative-hypnotic, or anxiolytic abuse (Miller, 1991). Approximately 15% of individuals with alcohol use disorders develop clinical depressions (Schuckit, 1986), and over half have significant symptoms of anxiety (Smail, Stockwell, Canter & Hodgson, 1984). In the elderly, alcohol use disorders are present in at least 15% of older patients seen by psychiatrists for psychiatric disorders ranging from depression to acute psychotic states (Schuckit, 1982). The differential diagnosis of comorbid depression or other psychiatric disorders should include dementia, which is an important complication in elderly who chronically abuse alcohol, sedative-hypnotic, anxiolytic, anticholinergic, or antihistaminic agents (Blazer, 1989).

Evaluation of the elderly person at risk for substance abuse and psychiatric illness should start with a thorough psychiatric, medical and social history. Direct inquiry regarding the frequency and quantity of alcohol and drug use may be useful (including prescribed medications and over-the-counter preparations), as reports of even minor use may be significant. Total use may be underestimated due to denial or memory impairment, and even small amounts of alcohol or drugs may have serious adverse effects. Corroborative history by family members or care providers is especially helpful. In addition to information about patterns of use and changes in behavior, suspicious injuries and episodes of confusion should also be solicited from the patient and family. When individuals live alone or have no available family members, identification of elderly individuals with psychiatric or substance-related problems may occur by training public service and residential service workers to identify and refer isolated elderly who are at risk (Jinks & Raschko, 1990).

The major consequences of alcohol and other substance use disorders in the elderly are psychiatric and medical complications (Miller, 1991). A summary of important cues to substance abuse in the elderly may be recalled by the mnemonic SIMPLE: S = Seizures; I = Injuries or falls; M = Malnutrition and muscle wasting; P = Poor hygiene and self-neglect; L = Liver function abnormalities; E = Emotional and cognitive changes including lability, confusion, memory changes and unusual behavior.

Treatment

Mental health professionals and substance abuse counselors seldom receive adequate training in the mental health and medical needs of the elderly (Schuckit, 1982). Similarly, mental health care providers are often inexperienced in substance abuse treatment, and substance abuse treatment providers are often inexperienced in the treatment of severe mental illness (Ridgely, Goldman & Willenbring, 1990). Treatment modifications are necessary that consider the different needs of individuals with dual disorders, as well as the specialized needs of the elderly individual. As there are no empirical data on the comparative efficacy of various treatment models for dual disorders in the elderly, the authors suggest practical considerations and potential pitfalls in treatment. These approaches are not intended to be treatment guidelines, but instead suggest possible directions for further development. Two approaches to treatment have been chosen for discussion, each preceded by a case illustration. The first describes traditional substance abuse services modified for elderly individuals with acute, comorbid affective and anxiety disorders. The second approach

describes an integrated model of treatment for dual disorders adapted
to elderly individuals with persistent psychotic mental disorders.

SUBSTANCE ABUSE SERVICES ADAPTED FOR ELDERLY
WITH ACUTE PSYCHIATRIC DISORDERS

Case Vignette:

> Mrs. Y is a 71 year old woman who enjoyed an active life with good
> emotional and physical health until age 65. She had used alcohol
> socially but had no previous problems associated with her alcohol
> use. At 65, with symptoms of decreased visual acuity, she was diag-
> nosed with adult onset diabetes mellitus that eventually required in-
> sulin management. Shortly after this diagnosis she complained to her
> internist of insomnia that was treated with low doses of lorazepam.
> Mrs. Y's husband of 45 years died one year ago. Since his death, she
> became more socially isolative, began using "slightly more" alcohol,
> and experienced a reemergence of the insomnia. In addition, she was
> observed by her internist and daughter to be more anxious, requiring
> larger doses of lorazepam to manage her symptoms. She had inter-
> mittent periods of confusion and forgetfulness, and required two
> hospitalizations in the last year for diabetic ketoacidosis associated
> with poor compliance with diet and insulin administration. Most
> recently she began complaining of severe pain in her legs, arms,
> chest, and head. She began to obsess about her physical condition and
> took increasing doses of lorazepam, either "borrowing" it from neigh-
> bors or getting additional medication prescribed by her internist.
> Referrals to a series of medical specialists consistently concluded that
> there was no acute medical illness accounting for her symptoms.
> Despite these consultations and second opinions, Mrs. Y persisted in
> the belief that her problems were physical.
> Mrs. Y's increasing tolerance to the effects of lorazepam, her in-
> creased use of alcohol, and deteriorating level of function, culminated
> in a consulting psychiatrist's diagnosis of minor tranquilizer and al-
> cohol dependence. A history of several losses and marked somatic
> symptoms, coupled with insomnia and anxiety also pointed to the
> strong possibility of an underlying affective disorder.
> In a family session Mrs. Y's daughter and son were able to convince
> Mrs. Y to be admitted to the psychiatric unit of a general hospital.
> During the early phase of the admission she was detoxified from
> alcohol and lorazepam, and control of her diabetes mellitus was rees-
> tablished. After stabilization of her withdrawal symptoms she con-

tinued to exhibit marked obsessional behavior focusing on her "physical" pain. Antidepressant management with paroxetine was initiated with significant resolution of depressive symptoms in three weeks. The episodes of confusion and memory impairment similarly resolved. Discharge planning included follow-up with a geropsychiatrist who would coordinate Mrs. Y's psychiatric and medical care, referral to a community senior center which has senior AA meetings every day, and placement with her daughter at her daughter's home.

This case illustrates many of the challenges of identifying and treating overlapping symptoms from concurrent substance abuse, psychiatric illness, and medical illness in an elderly individual. Mrs. Y's reported consumption of modest amounts of alcohol, use of prescribed medications for symptoms of anxiety, and active medical problems made assessment of her anxiety and depressive symptoms difficult. Her insistence on a medical diagnosis as the cause of her unexplained symptoms resulted in numerous medical evaluations that failed to detect her problem of substance abuse, while her internist unknowingly contributed to her problems by increasing her access to drugs. The recent loss of her spouse, combined with declining health are common events associated with aging and overshadowed substance abuse as a possible reason for changes in mood, function, and behavior. These same stressors are risk factors for the development of late-onset substance abuse in the elderly who have a history of routine moderate drinking or anxiolytic use (Finney & Moos, 1984). Mrs. Y's episodes of confusion and forgetfulness were also important clues of chronic alcohol and benzodiazepine abuse, yet there were several other possible causes including metabolic derangements from poor diabetic control, early signs of dementia (contributing to treatment noncompliance), and impaired cognition (pseudodementia) secondary to major depression.

These interrelated symptoms and disorders required concurrent assessment and treatment. Mrs. Y's treatment began with the mobilization of family support and admission for acute stabilization of her diabetes and detoxification from her alcohol and prescription drug dependence. This allowed for better assessment of her psychological symptoms resulting in eventual treatment of a concurrent major depression.

Approaches to treatment vary with individual needs and the types of substances abused. The increased risk of cognitive impairment and medical problems in the elderly dictate that an essential part of treatment is a thorough cognitive, neurological, and medical evaluation. The dually diagnosed elderly patient who is difficult to engage in an outpatient evaluation may require brief inpatient hospitalization to provide a medical assessment, to safely conduct chemical detoxification, and to initiate acute treatment of psychiatric and substance abuse symptoms. During the acute phase of management, aggressive treatment of active medical problems is warranted in conjunction with an assessment of possible medication side effects and drug interactions. Ideally, attempts should be made to minimize polypharmacy and to discontinue all unnecessary agents.

Some individuals with alcohol use disorders may be successfully treated by primary clinicians on an outpatient basis including emotional support, medical care, and referral to socialization groups. Adjunctive treatments such as disulfram, low dose antidepressants, and methadone may be used effectively in the elderly following careful pretreatment assessment and close medical supervision (Atkinson & Kofoed, 1984). Outpatient benzodiazepine withdrawal programs may be better tolerated by the elderly who tend to have less severe withdrawal symptoms compared to younger patients (Schweizer, Case & Rickel, 1989). Outpatient approaches are especially appropriate for individuals with late-onset alcohol disorders who tend to have high treatment compliance (Atkinson & Kofoed, 1984). Multidisciplinary treatment teams that emphasize outreach and social support have also been successful models of treatment (Bissell & Sweeney, 1981). Long-term treatment of the substance use disorders may include 12-step, self-help programs such as Alcoholics Anonymous or Narcotics Anonymous, but some socially restrained elderly individuals do not find these groups compatible due to the candid and sometimes profane self-disclosures and younger age composition (Atkinson & Kofoed, 1984). Some studies of elderly alcohol users suggest that age-specific groups for the elderly may be more beneficial than mixed-age groups (Kofoed, Kania, Walsh & Atkinson, 1986).

Long-term treatment also requires maximal provision of social supports to counteract the isolation and withdrawal that frequently accompanies substance use disorders and psychiatric illness in the elderly. Family support and involvement (if available) should be an integrated part of treatment. Housing instability and homelessness are common complications of dual disorders (Drake & Wallach,

1989), suggesting that safe, stable, long-term housing is an important requisite to successful treatment. However, elderly patients may require additional support services specific to their cognitive and physical abilities. A systematic and thorough assessment of the elderly person's ability to conduct basic self-care and other activities of daily living may be necessary to assess the appropriate level of residential support services or setting, including the need for ongoing supervision of medical problems or long-term care placement.

INTEGRATED SUBSTANCE ABUSE TREATMENT FOR SEVERELY MENTALLY ILL ELDERLY

Acute affective and anxiety disorders are among the most likely comorbid psychiatric conditions associated with alcohol and other drug abuse in the elderly. However, the high prevalence of substance use among severely mentally ill younger and middle-aged adults, suggests that this cohort may present a growing challenge in older age. The following case exemplifies the different needs and problems associated with this subgroup.

Case Vignette:

Mr. K is a 66 year old man with schizoaffective disorder and a long-standing history of alcohol abuse. Over the years he has had multiple psychiatric hospitalizations for acute psychotic decompensations, as well as several brief inpatient detoxification admissions. During periods when he is not drinking and compliant with his prescribed medications (haloperidol, lithium, cardiazem, and synthroid), he continues to have mild paranoid symptoms and auditory hallucinations, yet he is able to maintain stable housing. On resuming drinking, he discontinues his medications and shortly develops grandiose delusions marked by belligerent, irritable, and hostile behaviors. These relapses into alcohol abuse have become more frequent over the last few years, resulting in multiple evictions from housing settings due to his destruction of property. His sister states that she does not want anything to do with him, yet she believes that he is becoming progressively more impaired in his judgment and that "he may be developing Alzheimer's Disease," yet Alzheimer's homecare services have been refused due to the primary diagnoses of severe mental illness and alcohol abuse.

Past attempts to arrange inpatient detoxification and substance abuse treatment have resulted in refusals to accept Mr. K with the prerequisite that his psychotic disorder be treated first. In the few instances when admission has occurred, Mr. K has signed out of the hospital within several days against medical advice. Outpatient treatment referrals have also been unsuccessful. Mr. K's delusional and belligerent behavior was not well-tolerated by the local Alcoholic's Anonymous meeting's participants. Furthermore, Mr. K is likely to become more agitated and paranoid when he attends large group meetings.

Mr. K's case manager became increasingly concerned that Mr. K had developed a persistent cough, shortness of breath, and fatigue. Mr. K at first refused a medical and psychiatric evaluation. Yet the case manager was persistent in pursuing attempts to engage Mr. K in treatment and suggested that housing could be arranged in a group home for elderly patients from the community mental health center, provided that he comply with the required pre-admission medical evaluation. As Mr. K was in temporary housing and at risk of eviction, he consented to the evaluation which ruled out tuberculosis and pneumonia, yet confirmed mild congestive heart failure, complicated by untreated hypothyroidism and symptoms of mild to moderate cognitive impairment.

Following treatment for these medical disorders and placement in an elderly group home, a case manager from a local community mental health center geriatric team with training in substance abuse was assigned to Mr. K with the plan to engage Mr. K in psychoeducational dual diagnosis treatment groups. Mr. K was placed on intramuscular haloperidol in conjunction with frequent lithium levels to assure medication compliance. Mr. K's cognition improved with supervised compliance on his medications, abstinence from alcohol, and correction of his hypothyroidism, ultimately facilitating his increasing participation in the dual diagnosis treatment program at the community mental health center.

This case illustrates the failure of traditional approaches to substance abuse treatment for severely mentally ill elderly. Reasons for failure include the unsuccessful attempt by several services with different orientations and mandates to provide care. This case study also shows the successful use of an integrated, concurrent, and comprehensive approach to psychiatric and substance abuse disorders. In addition, the importance of residential and medical needs are illustrated. Mr. K's capacity to participate in treatment are directly facilitated by specialized residential services for elderly mentally ill persons and successful management of medical problems affecting his function and cognition.

Outcomes for treatment of the elderly with dual diagnoses of severe mental illness and substance use disorder are unknown. However, innovative models for treatment of dual disorders have been described for younger age groups and are discussed elsewhere in the volume (Fariello & Scheidt, 1989; Minkoff & Drake, 1991) and shared features have emerged that may be relevant to treatment of the elderly. Key principles include the need for treatment to be integrated, concurrent, in the same setting, and provided by clinicians who are cross-trained in substance use disorders and severe mental illness.

Some of the problems associated with traditional approaches to dual diagnosis treatment are likely to be compounded in the elderly. The elderly are especially vulnerable to fragmented, overlapping, and sometimes conflicting services by multiple providers with different treatment philosophies. For example, the elderly dually diagnosed individual may receive services from several different medical specialists, a psychiatrist, elder case workers, mental health case managers, homemakers, visiting nurses, respite care workers, substance abuse clinicians, and may also attend 12-step, self-help groups and senior citizen center programs. This fragmentation of providers may facilitate conflicting treatment approaches, poor coordination of services, and treatment noncompliance. In addition, multiple providers in different settings may invite prescription and other drug abuse by failing to centralize the necessary information to make an accurate diagnosis.

Additional problems in coordinating and financing services exist at the level of states where several agencies may be involved in services for the dually diagnosed elderly individual, including separate state administrations for elderly services, mental health services, alcohol and drug abuse services, and elder housing or long-term care facilities. The special needs of the elderly person with a substance use disorder and severe mental illness (and possible comorbid cognitive impairment) are likely to be lost among this daunting array of providers and systems. Designating a single clinician as responsible for coordinating resources is crucial, yet single providers such as primary care physicians or elder case managers seldom have extensive training in the treatment of severe mental illness or substance abuse.

The efficacy of 12-step, self-help groups for severely mentally ill elderly people is not known. Clinical experience in programs for younger individuals with psychotic disorders suggests that treatment is frequently unsuccessful when referrals are made to groups that are confrontational, abstinence-oriented, unsophisticated regarding the use of prescribed psychotropic medications, or unfamiliar with psychotic or delusional individuals. For these individuals, alternative approaches emphasize engaging the individual in treatment through assertive case management, through facilitating the acquisition of basic needs such as housing and entitlements, and through group treatment that is psychoeducational and behavioral in orientation (Drake, Bartels, Teague, Noordsy & Clark, 1993; Minkoff & Drake, 1991). These approaches may be more appropriate than traditional substance abuse treatment options for the substance abusing elderly individual with psychotic mental illness or cognitive impairment.

Vocational rehabilitation and family involvement are key components of a comprehensive approach to younger dually diagnosed individuals, yet these factors may be different in the treatment of the older individual. Full-time, paid employment may not be a common goal for the elderly dually diagnosed person. Rehabilitation approaches may be useful to develop social skills and behaviors in order to successfully remain in elderly congregate living settings, or to participate in senior center and other leisure activities. Similarly, the elderly dually diagnosed person may no longer have family who are in proximity or involved in their care. Instead, residential support services and psychoeducational approaches may be necessary for surrogate family members, including live-in companions or group home caretakers. In those instances when family members are available and involved, they are likely to be siblings, spouses, or adult children. These individuals may require respite or other homecare services to maintain their elderly family member at home, as well as assistance in finding appropriate alternative group home or long-term care settings.

CONCLUSION

Many basic questions remain unanswered about dual diagnosis in the elderly. A first priority for investigation should be a systematic study of the prevalence and correlates of comorbid psychiatric and substance use disorders in the elderly. Demographic studies are needed that use standardized instruments to describe the extent of the problem and to identify risk factors and characteristics. Subgroups within dually diagnosed populations need to be identified and described with the goal of determining appropriate diagnostic and treatment approaches. For example, individuals who have an alcohol use disorder are likely to have characteristics and treatment needs that are different, depending on the separate comorbid psychiatric diagnoses of depression, schizophrenia, or dementia. Similarly, late-onset substance abuse and psychiatric disorders require further study with comparisons to chronic or life-long disorders. Longitudinal studies with long-term follow-up periods are needed to define the natural history of dual diagnosis and to assess outcomes. Prospective, randomized studies are also needed to determine effective treatment options. Finally, services research will be important to test different models and systems of health care delivery with respect to outcomes and cost.

REFERENCES

Abernethy, D. (1992). Psychotropic drugs and the aging process: Pharmacokinetics and pharmacodynamics. In C. Salzman (Ed.), *Clinical Geriatric Psychopharmacology.* (pp. 61–76). Baltimore: Williams and Wilkins.

Ananth, J., Vandewater, S., Kamal, M., Brodsky, A., Gamal, R., & Miller, M. (1989). Missed diagnosis of substance abuse in psychiatric patients. *Hospital and Community Psychiatry. 40,* 297–299.

Atkinson, R. M., & Kofoed, L. L. (1984). Alcohol and Drug Abuse. In C.K. Cassel & J.R. Walsh (Eds.) *Geriatric Medicine.* (pp. 219–235). New York: Springer-Verlag.

Bartels, S. J., Drake, R. E., & Wallach, M.A. (1995). The long-term course of substance abuse in people with severe mental illness. *Psychiatric Services. 46,* 248–251.

Beardsley, R. S, Gardocki, G. L., Larson, D. B., & Hidalgo, J. (1988). Prescribing of psychotropic medications by primary care physicians and psychiatrists. *Archives of General Psychiatry. 45*, 1117–1119.

Beresford, T. P., Blow, F. C., Bower, K. J., Adams, K., & Hall, R.C. (1988). Alcoholism and aging in the general hospital. *Psychosomatics. 29*, 61–72.

Bissell, L., & Sweeney, G. (1981). Alcoholism outreach to single room occupancies. *American Journal of Drug and Alcohol Abuse. 8*, 215–224.

Blazer, D. G. (1989). Alcohol and drug problems in the elderly. In E.W. Busse, & D.G. Blazer (Eds.) *Geriatric Psychiatry.* (pp. 489–511). Washington, DC: American Psychiatric Press, Inc.

Blazer, D., & Williams C. D. (1980). Epidemiology of dysphoria and depression in an elderly population. *American Journal of Psychiatry. 137*(4), 439–444.

Cohen, C. I., Teresi, J., & Holmes, D. (1988). The mental health of old homeless men. *Journal of American Geriatric Society. 36*, 492–501.

Cook, B., Winokur, G., Garvey, M., & Beach, V. (1991). Depression and previous alcoholism in the elderly. *British Journal of Psychiatry. 158*, 72–75.

Curtis, J. R., Geller, G., Stokes, E. J., Levine, D.M., & Moore, R.D. (1989). Characteristics, diagnosis, and treatment of alcoholism in elderly patients. *Journal of the American Geriatrics Society. 37*:310–316.

Drake, R. E., Bartels, S. J., Teague, G. B., Noordsy, D. L., & Clark, R. E. (1993). Treatment of substance abuse in severely mentally ill patients. *Journal of Nervous and Mental Disease. 181*, 606–611.

Drake, R. E., Osher F.C., & Wallach, M. A. (1989). Alcohol use and abuse in schizophrenia: a prospective study. *Journal of Nervous and Mental Disease. 177*, 408–414.

Drake, R. E., & Wallach, M. A. (1989). Substance abuse among the chronically mentally ill. *Hospital and Community Psychiatry. 40*, 1041–1046.

Fariello, D., & Scheidt, S. (1989). Clinical case management of the dually diagnosed patient. *Hospital and Community Psychiatry, 40*, 1065–1067.

Finlayson, R., Hurt, R., Lavis, L.J., & Morse, R.M. (1988). Alcoholism in elderly persons: A study of the psychiatric and psychosocial features of 216 patients. *Mayo Clinic Proceedings. 63*, 761–768.

Finney, J. W., & Moos, R. H. (1984). Life stressors and problem drinking among older adults. *Recent Developments in Alcoholism. 2*, 267–288.

Hasin, D.S., Endicott, J., & Keller, M.B. (1991). Alcohol problems in Psychiatric patients: 5-year course. *Comprehensive Psychiatry. 32*(4), 303–316.

Jinks, M. J., & Raschko, R. (1990). A profile of alcohol and prescription drug abuse in a high-risk community-based elderly population. *The Annals of Pharmacotherapy. 24*(10), 971–975.

Kofoed, L. L., Kania, J., Walsh, T., & Atkinson, R. (1986). Outpatient treatment of patients with substance abuse and coexisting psychiatric disorders. *American Journal of Psychiatry. 143*(7), 867–872.

Krystal, J. H., Leaf, P. J., Bruce, M. L., & Charney, D. S. (1992). Effects of age and alcoholism on the prevalence of panic disorder. *Acta Psychiatrica Scandinavica. 85,* 77–82.

Loosen, P. T., Dew, B. W., & Prange, A. J. (1990). Long-term predictors of outcome in abstinent alcoholic men. *American Journal of Psychiatry. 147,* 1662–1666.

Miller, N. S. (1991). Alcohol and drug dependence. In J. Sadavoy, L.W. Lazarus & L.F. Jarvik (Eds.) *Comprehensive Review of Geriatric Psychiatry.* (pp. 387–401). Washington, DC: American Psychiatric Press, Inc.

Minkoff, K., & Drake, R. E. (1991). *Dual Diagnosis of Major Mental Illness and Substance Disorder.* San Francisco: Jossey-Bass.

Myers, J. K., Weissman, M. M., Tischler, G L., Holzer, C. E., Leaf, P. J., Orvaschel, H., Anthony, J. C., Boyd, J. H., Burke, J. D., Kramer, M., & Stoltzman, R. (1984): Six-month prevalence of psychiatric disorders in three communities. *Archives of General Psychiatry. 41,* 959–970.

Palinkas, L. A., Wingard, D. L., & Barrett-Connor, E. (1990). Chronic illness and depressive symptoms in the elderly: A population-based study. *Journal of Clinical Epidemiology. 43*(11), 1131–1141.

Ridgely, M., Goldman, H., & Willenbring, M. (1990). Barriers to the care of persons with dual diagnoses: Organizational and financing issues. *Schizophrenia Bulletin. 16,* 123–132.

Robins, L. N., Helzer, J.E., & Przybeck, T. R. (1988). Alcohol disorders in the community: A report from the Epidemiologic Catchment Area. In R. Ross, J. Barrett (Eds.) *Alcoholism: Origins and Outcome.* 15–29.

Schuckit, M.A. (1982). A clinical review of alcohol, alcoholism and the elderly patient. *Journal of Clinical Psychiatry. 43*(10), 396–399.

Schuckit, M.A. (1986). Genetic and clinical implications of alcoholism and affective disorder. *American Journal of Psychiatry. 143:* 140–147.

Schweizer, E., Case, G., & Rickels, K. (1989). Benzodiazepine dependence and withdrawal in elderly patients. *American Journal of Psychiatry. 146*(4), 529–531.

Smail, P., Stockwell, T., Canter S., & Hodgson, R. (1984). Alcohol dependence and phobic anxiety states, I: a prevalence study. *British Journal of Psychiatry. 144,* 529–531.

Speer, D., & Bates, K. (1992). Comorbid mental and substance disorders among older psychiatric patients. *Journal of the American Geriatric Society. 40,* 886–890.

Spencer, G. (1989). Projections of the population of the United States, by age, sex and race: 1988 to 2080. Series P-25, No 1018 Washington, DC, U.S. Department of Commerce.

Tarter, R., & Ryan, C. (1983). Neuropsychology of alcoholism: Etiology, phenomenology, process, and outcome. In M. Galenter (Eds.), *Recent Developments in Alcoholism* New York: Plenum.

Turner, W. M., & Tsuang, M. T. (1990). Impact of substance abuse on the course and outcome of schizophrenia. *Schizophrenia Bulletin. 16*, 87–95.

Vaillant, G. E. (1983). *The Natural History of Alcoholism.* Cambridge, MA: Harvard University Press.

Whitcup, S., & Miller, F. (1987). Unrecognized drug dependence in psychiatrically hospitalized elderly patients. *The American Geriatrics Society. 35*(4), 297–301.

Zimberg, S. (1987). Alcohol abuse among the elderly. In L.L. Carstensen & B.A. Edelstein (Eds), *Handbook of Clinical Gerontology* (pp. 57–65). New York: Pergamon Press.

Zisook, S., Heaton, R., Mornaville, J., Kuck, J., Jernigan, T., & Braff D. (1992). Past substance abuse and clinical course of schizophrenia. *American Journal of Psychiatry. 149*: 552–553.

NOTE

Preparation of this chapter was supported by NIMH Geratric Clinical Mental Health Academic Award 1K07MH01052.

10

HIV, Substance Abuse, and Mental Illness

JOHN C. MAHLER

INTRODUCTION

HIV infection is a significant and growing problem among persons
with chronic mental illness and substance abuse disorders. Few
patients present a greater challenge to the knowledge, skills, and
professional commitment of the clinician. From initial assessment to
closure of treatment, crucial questions and issues emerge where little,
if any, empirical data exist. Differential diagnosis and treatment planning require expertise in medical disorders, psychopathology,
psychopharmacology, and psychosocial treatments. Yet, with careful
diagnostic and treatment practices, working with these individuals
can be remarkably rewarding. This chapter will first present basic information about HIV that is essential for any mental health or substance abuse provider. It then covers the scope of the HIV problem in
persons with chronic mental illness and substance abuse disorders
and discusses specific prevention and treatment considerations for
dually diagnosed persons.

HUMAN IMMUNODEFICIENCY VIRUS

Historical Background

In the summer of 1981 the Center for Disease Control (CDC) reported the unexplained occurrence of 5 cases of Pneumocystis carinii pneumonia (PCP) and 26 cases of Kaposi's sarcoma (KS) in previously healthy homosexual men. Reports of PCP in intravenous drug abusers quickly followed, and by year end more than 300 adults had succumbed to the mysterious and ultimately fatal syndrome. In 1982, analysis of an additional 1000 cases suggested a transmissible agent was the likely cause and the syndrome became known as the acquired immunodeficiency syndrome (AIDS). In the following year AIDS would be reported in recipients of blood transfusions and blood products (hemophiliacs), heterosexual partners of intravenous drug abusers and hemophiliacs, as well as infants of infected mothers. It was not until 1984 that the etiologic agent was identified as a retrovirus which ultimately would be called Human Immunodeficiency Virus (HIV). By the end of 1985, reliable tests for antibodies to HIV were widely available. The availability of this test reassured the public about the safety of the blood supply, but this was quickly followed by the recognition that more than 1 million people were infected in the United States and approximately 10 million people were infected worldwide.

Diagnostic Classification

The case definition of AIDS and the classification of clinical stages of HIV infection have undergone several revisions over the years to reflect emerging scientific findings and changes in clinical practice. Table 10.1 is the 1993 Revised Classification System for HIV Infection including the updated AIDS case definition. With this revised AIDS case definition, patients may meet the AIDS case definition by either of two criteria: a CD4+ count of less than 200 or CD4+ percentage of less than 14; or a Category C clinical condition.

Transmission

Transmission of HIV occurs only when cells containing viral particles enter into the bloodstream. Cells containing infectious material are found most abundantly in blood, but are also present in significant quantities in semen and cervical secretions, and in low concentrations in tears and perspiration. However, there is no evidence of transmission by casual contact.

Worldwide the major mode of transmission is heterosexual intercourse, which accounts for 75–85% of cases. The rate of risk for each exposure and for each type of behavior is not precisely known, nor is it known why some individuals do not become infected despite repeated exposures. However, risk of infection is known to increase with a greater number of partners, with receptive anal intercourse, with failure to use condoms, and with practices that promote rectal tearing. Coexisting genital ulcers, greater immunosuppression in the infected partner, and a history of sexually transmitted diseases are also related to enhanced sexual transmission. Male to male and male to female transmission are more easily accomplished than female to male transmission, but as the number of infected women increases, female to male transmission will become more prevalent.

The virus is also efficiently transmitted by blood or blood products both in individuals who share contaminated needles for injection drug use and in those who receive transfusions of blood or blood products. Again, the precise risk for an individual injection drug user is unknown, but the duration of use, the frequency of sharing, the number of individuals sharing the apparatus, the location of use (e.g., shooting gallery), and the prevalence of HIV in the intravenous drug using (IDU) community affect the risk of transmission. The risk of becoming infected by blood transfusion has significantly declined since the introduction of HIV-1 antibody testing (Centers for Disease Control and Prevention, 1990).

Neuropsychiatric Syndromes of AIDS

Neuropsychiatric complications occur commonly during the course of HIV infection. Because the clinical presentations and differential diagnosis differ between early HIV infection and AIDS, establishing the stage of HIV infection by history (CDC classification) and CD4+ T cell count is the first step to diagnosis.

Although less common than in the late stages of HIV infection, neuropsychiatric presentations have been reported in the early phases of HIV infection including both primary infection and seroconversion (Perry, 1990-b). Early in the HIV epidemic, case reports described focal and diffuse encephalopathies, ataxia, and

Table 10.1. 1993 Revised Classification System for HIV Infection
(Source: Centers for Disease Control and Prevention (1993))

Clinical Categories

Category A

Category A consists of one or more of the conditions listed below in an adolescent or adult (≥ 13 years) with documented HIV infection. Conditions listed in Categories B and C must not have occurred.

- Asymptomatic HIV infection
- Persistent generalized lymphadenopathy
- Acute (primary) HIV infection with accompanying illness or history of acute HIV infection

Category B

Category B consists of symptomatic conditions in an HIV-infected adolescent or adult that are not included among conditions listed in clinical Category C and that meet at least one of the following criteria: a) the conditions are attributed to HIV infection or are indicative of a defect in cell-mediated immunity; or b) the conditions are considered by physicians to have a clinical course or to require management that is complicated by HIV infection. Examples of conditions in clinical Category B include, but are not limited to:

- Bacillary angiomatosis
- Candidiasis, oropharyngeal (thrush)
- Candidiasis, vulvovaginal; persistent, frequent, or poorly responsive to therapy
- Cervical dysplasia (moderate or severe)/cervical carcinoma in situ
- Constitutional symptoms, such as fever (38.5°C) or diarrhea lasting >1 month
- Hairy luekoplakia, oral
- Herpes zoster (shingles), involving at least two distinct episodes or more than one dermatome
- Idiopathic thrombocytopenic purpura
- Listeriosis
- Pelvic inflammatory disease, particularly if complicated by tubo-ovarian abscess
- Peripheral neuropathy

For classification purposes, Category B conditions take precedence over those in Category A. For example, someone previously treated for oral or persistent vaginal candidiasis (and who has not developed a Category C disease) but who is now asymptomatic should be classified in clinical Category B.

cont'd

Category C

Category C includes the clinical conditions listed in the AIDS surveillance case definition. For classification purposes, once a Category C condition has occurred, the person will remain in Category C.

AIDS Surveillance Case Definition

- Candidiasis of bronchi, trachea, or lungs
- Candidiasis, esophageal
- Cervical cancer, invasive*
- Coccidiodomycosis, disseminated or extrapulmonary
- Cryptococcosis, extrapulmonary
- Cryptosporidiosis, chronic intestinal (>1 month's duration)
- Cytomegalovirus disease (other than liver, spleen, or nodes)
- Cytomegalovirus retinitis (with loss of vision)
- Encephalopathy, HIV-related
- Herpes simplex: chronic ulcer(s) (>1 month's duration); or bronchitis, pneumonitis, or esophagitis
- Histoplasmosis, disseminated or extrapulmonary
- Isosporiasis, chronic intestinal (>1 month's duration)
- Kaposi's sarcoma
- Lymphoma, Burkitt's (or equivalent term)
- Lymphoma, primary, of brain
- Mycobacterium avium complex or M. kansasii, disseminated or extrapulmonary
- Mycobacterium tuberculosis, any site (pulmonary* or extrapulmonary)
- Mycobacterium, other species or unidentified species, disseminated or extrapulmonary
- Pneumocystis carinii pneumonia
- Pneumonia, recurrent*
- Progressive multifocal leukoencephalopathy
- Salmonella septicemia, recurrent
- Toxoplasmosis of brain
- Wasting syndrome due to HIV

*(Added in the 1993 expansion of the AIDS surveillance case definition.)

CD4+ T-Lymphocyte Categories

	CD4+ T-Cells/µL	CD4+ Percentage (%)
Category 1	≥500	≥29
Category 2	200–499	14–28
Category 3	<200	<14

The lowest accurate, but not necessarily the most recent, CD4+ T-lymphocyte count should be used for classification purposes.

meningitis presenting either within the context of the HIV seroconversion reaction or with minimal associated systemic symptoms. These conditions appeared to develop abruptly, to be time limited, and to be followed by a good and usually complete recovery. Deficits seen in early HIV infection in persons with chronic mental illness and substance abuse must be considered in clinical context since the effects of alcohol or drugs on neuropsychiatric performance may be similar to those described in early HIV infection (Perry, 1990-a).

Neuropsychiatric deficits seen in late HIV infection are often due to the organic effects of HIV and associated conditions in the brain, but can be further complicated by alcohol/drug abuse and mental disorders. AIDS patients are vulnerable to a wide range of pathological conditions which affect the brain, including opportunistic infections, opportunistic neoplasms, the direct neurotoxic effects of HIV infection itself, and metabolic disturbances which accompany severe medical illnesses. As a result most patients with AIDS develop one of the HIV associated organic mental disorders prior to their death, including headache, meningitis, focal neurological symptoms, seizures, delirium and dementia.

EXTENT OF THE HIV PROBLEM IN PERSONS WITH CHRONIC MENTAL ILLNESS AND SUBSTANCE ABUSE DISORDERS

Efforts to determine the effect of the HIV epidemic on patients with mental disorders and substance abuse have just begun to define its extent of the problem in this patient population. Anonymous serological surveys of patients admitted to psychiatric hospitals in New York City have found rates of HIV infection ranging from 5.5% to 14.4% (Cournos et al., 1991; Empfield et al., 1993; Lee, Travin & Blueston, 1992: Sacks, Dermatis, Looser-Ott & Perry, 1992; Volavka, Convit, Czobor, Douyon, O'Donnell & Ventura, 1991). Abstinence-based alcohol and drug treatment programs have been less well studied, but seroprevalence rates of 10.3% to 13.3% have been reported (Jacobson, Worner, Sacks & Liebet, 1990; Mahler, Perry, Yi, Sacks & Dermatis, 1993).

The elevated rates of HIV infection in psychiatric and alcohol/drug treatment populations have been only partially explained. In all of these studies, history of injection drug use was strongly associated with seropositivity. The majority of these studies also found significant associations with male homosexual behavior, and one study reported an association with high risk heterosexual behaviors. Future research on correlates of HIV transmission will need to utilize improved methodologies such as link-file systems. This method allows the results of serological testing to be *linked* with the results of subject interviews about high risk behaviors such that the anonymity of both procedures is maintained. Further, new perspectives such as social network theory will also better inform the effort to understand HIV transmission in this vulnerable population.

Studies of HIV-related *risk behaviors* in patients with dual disorders show that a significant proportion of these individuals are at risk for developing HIV. Careful surveys of the behaviors of both inpatient and outpatient psychiatric patients reveal that close to half or more are sexually active, and that significant minorities of patients have unprotected sexual activities with multiple partners, have had a sexually transmitted infection, have exchanged sex for money or drugs, have unprotected anal intercourse, and/or have engaged in intravenous drug use (Sacks, Perry, Graver & Shindledecker, 1990; Kelly et al., 1992; Kalichman, Kelly, Johnson & Bulto, 1994, Cournos et al., 1994). Kalichman and colleagues (1994) found that over one-third of 95 chronically mentally ill patients they surveyed had two or more risk factors for HIV. Clinicians may find these data surprising since persons with chronic mental illness tend to be viewed as asexual by many mental health workers.

Associations between specific psychiatric disorders and risk behaviors have been found including associations between increased risk behavior and bipolar disorder, alcoholism, cocaine abuse, and antisocial personality disorder, as well as between reduced risk and schizophrenia, depressive disorders, and organic mental syndromes (Brooner, Greenfield, Schmidt & Bigelow, 1993; Schleifer & Keller 1991; Stiffman, Dore, Earls & Cunningham 1992). However, in a study of persons with schizophrenia, Cournos and colleagues (1994) found that 44% of patients had been sexually active in the preceding six months, and sexual activity was usually accompanied by HIV risk. Elevated rates of victimization among persons with chronic mental illness may also increase the risk of these individuals. The available evidence thus highlights the extent to which persons with chronic mental illness engage in behaviors putting them at risk for HIV infection and reinforces the need to develop effective interventions for risk reduction and prevention.

HIV RISK REDUCTION AND PREVENTION IN PERSONS WITH
CHRONIC MENTAL ILLNESS

Why do people change their health-related behaviors? Behaviors which are "well established, biologically driven, pleasurably reinforced, ego-syntonic, accompanied by high arousal states, and associated with distant rather than immediate threat" are more refractory to change (Perry, 1990-a). Among the models advanced for understanding and intervening with health behaviors, the health belief model fits well with the psychoeducational approach used with persons who have mental illness and substance abuse disorders. As described by Johnson, Ostrow and Joseph (1990), the health belief model posits that a "number of factors operate to either promote or retard desired behavior change: *knowledge* of health risks and health promoting behaviors, *perception* of oneself as being at risk and relating one's risk to one's actions, *perceived effectiveness* of behavior change and response efficacy, *belief* in the power of technological cures or preventions (e.g., faith that a vaccine to prevent HIV infection will soon be discovered), *sociodemographic variables* and *social network affiliation and group norms.*"

Research in patients with chronic mental illness has demonstrated that these individuals frequently lack accurate *knowledge* about HIV (Kelly et al., 1992; Hanson, Kramer, Gross, Quintana, Li & Asher, 1992; Baer, Dwyer & Lewitter-Koehler, 1988; Coverdale & Aruffo, 1992). Lacking specific educational models for teaching AIDS prevention to persons with chronic mental illness, studies have attempted to adapt educational programs originally developed for other populations. Three previous studies have shown increases in patients' knowledge after psychoeducational interventions (Lauer-Listhaus & Watterson, 1988; Sladyk, 1990; Goisman, Kent, Montgomery, Cheevers & Goldfinger, 1991); at least one such educational program failed to show any increase in patient knowledge about HIV (Cates & Graham, 1993). Although this research is still in its early phases, a consistent theme has been that simplicity and repetition with visual aids are probably essential to increase AIDS knowledge of dually diagnosed persons.

As reflected in the health belief model above, knowledge alone may not change behavior. McDermott, Sautter, Winstead and Quirk (1994) surveyed a group of acute psychiatric inpatients and controls to determine how HIV-related health beliefs and knowledge predicted changes in high-risk behaviors. They found that persons with schizophrenia differed from control subjects in that knowledge about HIV infection and AIDS did *not* change behavior. Patients with schizophrenia "appeared willing to change their behavior only if they believed their behavior could really make a difference in whether they would become infected" (McDermott et al., 1994). These beliefs need to be addressed in developing AIDS prevention programs for persons with chronic mental illness.

Researchers and clinicians wishing to design an AIDS prevention program may choose from a variety of conceptual frameworks, including the health belief model, the theory of reasoned action, or the AIDS risk reduction model. Although a complete discussion of the development and implementation of an intervention program is beyond the scope of this chapter, several key issues warrant mention and must be considered. (See Johnson et al. (1990) for a comprehensive review.)

First, the objectives of the educational program must be clearly defined. Conducting a *needs assessment* is crucial to ensure that the program is designed to address the specific issues encountered in the target audience. Second, the format for educational efforts must take into consideration the individual needs of the patient. Small groups, informal settings, and adjunctive individual counseling can be combined to create an effective intervention strategy. Third, HIV testing with counseling should be available on site and integrated into ongoing treatment for the individual patient when appropriate. Fourth, the message must be tailored to meet the cognitive and emotional capacity of the patient. Fifth, sensitivity to the cultural background and language of the individual is important in developing the message and for patients with limited literacy skills, audiovisual and individual instruction are essential. Sixth, the selection of educators must recognize that trust and an ability to identify with the educator are keys to a successful program. Lastly, clarity, simplicity, and specificity define the effective message.

Treatment of psychopathology associated with HIV risk behaviors may also be an effective method for reducing risk behaviors. Drug treatment has produced significant risk reduction among intravenous drug users in methadone maintenance. The treatment of non-intravenous substance abuse and perhaps mental disorders associated with risk behaviors offer an appealing, though unproven approach to risk reduction. Finally, if we are expecting dually diagnosed persons to reduce their HIV risk, they need to be given the appropriate tools. Although controversial, supplying condoms to psychiatric in-patients and outpatients as well as clean needles to injection drug users may facilitate prevention. Mentally ill persons with substance abuse disorders may be too poor and impaired to obtain these materials without help.

TREATMENT ISSUES

HIV infection often makes the already difficult treatment of dually diagnosed persons even more challenging. Innovative treatment strategies discussed in other chapters of this volume including integrated mental health and substance abuse treatment with an outreach component become even more important to implement. Little is known about the effectiveness of specific treatment programs for HIV-infected dually diagnosed individuals. Special considerations around stress reduction, medical and psychiatric management around HIV infection are highlighted below.

Stress Reduction

Both the chronic, progressive, yet uncertain nature of HIV infection as well as the stigmatization of the disease and potential for transmission contribute to stress all people experience when learning that they are HIV positive. Clinicians may underestimate these stresses because of the frequent chaos in the lives of dually diagnosed individuals. A history of hospitalizations, homelessness and arrests does not make the knowledge of HIV infection any less frightening or devastating. Both exacerbations of preexisting psychopathology and new illnesses have been described. Dually diagnosed patients thus might have psychotic of affective relapses or worsening of substance abuse. Such relapses could compromise housing, lead to arrests or dropout from treatment. It is thus imperative to anticipate stress reactions to HIV testing. These will occur both in patients who deny or under-report risk factors and in patients who anticipate testing HIV positive.

First, patients must be reassured that their treating team will not abandon them and will provide emotional and concrete support to the extent possible. This will require that staff confront their own prejudices and fears about HIV. Further, patients need reassurance that the results of the testing are confidential. In certain patients, more formal psychoeducation, psychological based interventions such as stress prevention training, and pharmacotherapies are useful tools.

Anxiety, a frequent concomitant of chronic, progressive illness, may benefit from cognitive-behavioral psychotherapies and pharmacologic treatments with anxiolytic agents. Non-benzodiazepine anxiolytics such as buspirone are preferred because of their lower abuse liability in dually diagnosed people as well as the potential for memory impairment associated with benzodiazepine treatment.

The clinician facing the decision of whether to offer HIV counseling and testing to a patient with mental illness and drug abuse must carefully weigh the risks and benefits of this procedure in the context of the patient's current illness. Although the final decision to consent to testing rests with the patient, this does not release the clinician from responsibly pursuing the implications of testing for each patient. The following clinical example describes how a clinical team effectively managed the testing and counseling needs of a patient with a long history of poor coping responses.

Mary, a 43-year-old widowed Black woman, presented for inpatient alcohol/drug rehabilitation after her 17-year-old son threatened to leave unless she went for treatment. The previous evening, while intoxicated, Mary had threatened him with a razor when he attempted to throw out her crack and beer. Mary had a long history of paranoia, depression, and anxiety which antedated her alcohol/drug use, but which was significantly worsened by recent use of up to one case of beer and $100 of crack-cocaine per day.

She reported ten prior hospitalizations for detoxification and one prior inpatient rehabilitation. Although she denied any prior psychiatric treatment, she acknowledged a suicide attempt at age 12 in which she jumped out of a window and broke both her legs. Her alcohol/drug problems began at age 18 and included intravenous cocaine and heroin use intermittently until she stopped five years prior to admission.

Following admission, a prn Librium detoxification protocol was begun, but she did not require medication. She appeared guarded at times and was easily overwhelmed by affective material in the groups, having to leave at times due to intense anxiety or sadness. On two occasions she was administered lorazepam when she exited the group appearing quite anxious. However, by the second week of hospitalization, she did not require medication for agitation and was able to respond to staff interventions. Her guardedness and low frustration tolerance responded to a plan for developing new cognitive and behavioral skills, and expanding her social supports.

At the end of the second week of treatment she requested HIV testing because of concern about her past history of IDU. During pre-test counseling, she stated she preferred testing as an inpatient because of the supportive setting of the hospital, but she expressed concern about being ostracized by her peers if they were to learn that she was being tested. She discussed this concern initially in individual sessions and then in group therapy where she received considerable support from her peers. During the third week of her hospital stay she was informed that she had tested positive for antibodies to HIV-1. She responded to the news with sadness and concerns for herself and her family. However, she actively sought and received support from her boyfriend and family and then peers within the patient community. In the final week of hospitalization, she collaborated with the treatment team in developing a discharge plan which included an outpatient dual diagnosis day program, an HIV support group, and an HIV treatment center.

Medical Treatment

Disorganization, cognitive dysfunction, and other symptoms of chronic mental illness can lead to significant problems in the medical management of the HIV-infected dually diagnosed patient. Difficulties may appear in any aspect of treatment, including compliance with demanding medication regimens, attendance at appointments, and relationships with physicians and other medical personnel. Patients will often need additional support from psychiatric or substance abuse providers and encouragement to follow through with treatment recommendations. The mental health professional must also be willing to assume an active role in educating and consulting to the medical professionals involved in the care of these patients. Recognition of the patient's cognitive and emotional capacity, coping skills, and personal wishes early in the treatment process will facilitate the formation of an effective treatment alliance.

Mr. Y is a 35-year-old African-American man with a history of schizophrenia and intravenous drug abuse. His threatening behavior when psychotic and noncompliance with treatment resulted in his receiving essentially no outpatient services until, homeless, he was referred to an assertive outreach team. The team engaged Mr. Y by assisting him to obtain housing and working with his supportive mother who ensured that he received his biweekly injection of fluphenazine decanoate. Mr. Y learned during a past psychiatric hospitalization that he had a low white blood cell count, but refused HIV testing.

The team was able to persuade Mr. Y to obtain a medical checkup. In this more neutral setting, Mr. Y agreed to have the HIV test suggested by the primary care physician. When the team attempted to follow up on the results of the HIV test in order to provide support to the patient, it was discovered that the test results had been "lost." Unaccustomed to working with sometimes menacing chronically mental ill individuals, the medical clinic did not recognize the need to take responsibility for informing this individual of the results of his HIV test. It was clear that they were also inadequately prepared to provide appropriate counseling.

With proactive participation by the psychiatric team, the results were "located." The team then set up a medical appointment, was present when the positive result was given to the patient, provided additional counseling to the patient in the presence of the medical staff, and worked with the patient to obtain needed medications. The patient was very emphatic that he did not want his mother to know that he was infected with HIV, a request that the team assured him it would honor. He suffered a temporary relapse of his drug use after receiving his positive result, but restabilized back to his original baseline after a few weeks. The psychiatric team then accompanied the patient to all subsequent medical appointments.

Psychiatric Treatment

Psychiatric treatment of persons with HIV, chronic mental illness and substance abuse must be adjusted to account for both the psychological as well as biological impact of HIV infection of the patient. First, accurate diagnosis is critical. The dual diagnosis clinician is used to asking whether substance abuse or mental illness is the current cause of the patient's problem. Now, HIV-related problems must be considered. When attempting to distinguish between these possibilities, the clinician must frequently rely upon the psychological and physical symptoms that do not overlap. When evaluating a patient for depression, for example, fatigue and lethargy may be attributed to physical illness, but suicidal ideation and diurnal mood variation would increase the probability of diagnosing a mood disorder. In addition, other signs of systemic illness and a patient's subjective report that "this episode is different" will raise the index of suspicion for organic illness. When substance abuse complicates the presentation, the clinician must consider both acute intoxication states and withdrawal states. Lastly, iatrogenically induced disorders may result from the treatment of HIV infection and its medical complications. As a rule, symptoms should be considered to be organic in origin until proven otherwise. Similarly, alcohol- and drug-related disorders and iatrogenic syndromes should be considered before a functional diagnosis is made.

Psychopharmacologic approaches must consider both the stage of HIV disease and the presentation requiring treatment. Among the most common presentations that require pharmacologic treatment in non-dually diagnosed HIV-infected persons are sleep and pain disorders. The frequency with which these complaints occur in dually diagnosed persons is unknown. Aggressive treatment of sleep disturbances can produce improvement in quality of life and in cognitive functioning in patients where the additional impairment associated with sleep deprivation has produced dysfunction in a marginally compensated individual. Similarly, effective treatment of the pain associated with the sequelae of HIV disease can produce a reduction in associated anxiety and dysphoria. Concerns about the abuse liability of medications for the treatment of sleep and pain disorders can be addressed by using nonaddictive medications such as trazodone and by implementing protocols to control the patient's access to medication.

Persons infected with HIV appear to be more prone to the adverse side effects of neuroleptic agents, especially dystonia and neuroleptic malignant syndrome (Perry, 1990-b). Use of low potency neuroleptics may lead to fewer extrapyramidal side effects, but greater risk for cognitive impairment. Low potency neuroleptics should be avoided with focal presentations because of the potential for lowering seizure threshold. Benzodiazepines may be useful for acute management of agitation, but their effects on memory limit their utility for chronic symptoms. Selective serotonin reuptake inhibitors may be preferred to the heterocyclic antidepressants because of their lack of anticholinergic effects, but their effects on the metabolism of other medications must be considered.

Aggressive treatment of the brain must also be accompanied by appropriate treatment of the mind. Psychoeducation prior to the development of significant neuropsychiatric impairment prepares individuals to competently plan for their future. However, careful attention must be given to providing a realistic yet not hopeless picture of the future. As HIV disease progresses, intermittent, focused therapy for the individual and family will help each accept the series of losses that come with the patient's declining health. Crisis interventions may be needed when abrupt or unexpected changes occur. With this approach, both the patient and the family can emerge with a new sense of where to invest their interests and energies for the future.

CONCLUSION

Up to 15% of persons with chronic mental illness may suffer from HIV infection. Many more such patients are at risk for HIV due to high risk behaviors. Persons dually diagnosed with substance abuse are at increased risk for HIV. In spite of these worrisome epidemiologic data, little is known about how to prevent and treat HIV infection in person with chronic mental illness and substance abuse. Deficits in knowledge need to be corrected. Models of how to change health-related behaviors need to be developed and tested in dually diagnosed persons. For the moment, it is imperative that mental health, substance abuse and medical providers anticipate that all aspects of management of HIV in these individuals will require the utmost in sensitivity, support and attention to both the biological and psychological aspects of this devastating illness.

REFERENCES

Baer, J.W., Dwyer, P.C., & Lewitter-Koehler, S. (1988). Knowledge about AIDS Among Psychiatric Inpatients. *Hospital and Community Psychiatry. 39,* 986–988.

Brooner, R.K., Greenfield, L., Schmidt, C.W., & Bigelow, G.E. (1993). Antisocial Personality Disorder and HIV Infection Among Intravenous Drug Abusers. *American Journal of Psychiatry. 150*(1), 53–58.

Cates, J.A., & Graham, L.L. (1993). HIV and Serious Mental Illness: Reducing the Risk. *Community Mental Health Journal. 29,* 35–47.

Centers for Disease Control and Prevention. (1990). Estimates of HIV Prevalence and Projected AIDS Cases: Summary of a Workshop. *Morbidity and Mortality Weekly Report. 39,* 110–119.

Centers for Disease Control and Prevention. (1992). 1993 Revised Classification System for HIV Infection and Expanded Surveillance Case Definition for AIDS Among Adolescents and Adults. *Morbidity and Mortality Weekly Report. 41*(RR-17), 1–19.

Cournos, F., Empfield, M., Horwath, E., McKinnon, K., Meyer, I., Schrage, H., Currie, C., & Agosin, B. (1991). HIV Seroprevalence Among Patients Admitted to Two Psychiatric Hospitals. *American Journal of Psychiatry. 148*(9), 1225–1230.

Cournos, F., Guido, J.R., Coomaraswamy, S., Meyer-Bahlberg, H., Sugden, R., & Horvath, E. (1994). Sexual Activity and Risk of HIV infection Among Patients with Schizophrenia. *American Journal of Psychiatry. 151*,228–232.

Coverdale, J.H., & Aruffo, J.F. (1992). AIDS and Family Planning Counseling of Psychiatrically Ill Women in Community Mental Health Clinics. *Community Mental Health Journal. 28*, 13–20.

Empfield, M., Cournos, F., Meyer, I., McKinnon, K., Horwath, E., Silver, M., Schrage, H., & Herman, R. (1993). HIV Seroprevalence Among Homeless Patients Admitted to a Psychiatric Inpatient Unit. *American Journal of Psychiatry. 150*(1), 47–52.

Goisman, R.M., Kent, A.B., Montgomery, B.C., Cheevers, M.M., & Goldfinger, S.M. (1991). AIDS Education for Patients with Chronic Mental Illness. *Community Mental Health Journal. 27*, 189–197.

Hanson, M., Kramer, T.H., Gross, W., Quintana, J., Li, P.W., & Asher, R. (1992). AIDS Awareness and Risk Behaviors Among Dually Diagnosed Adults. *AIDS Education and Prevention. 4*, 41–51.

Jacobson, J.M., Worner, T.M., Sacks, H.S., & Liebet, C.S. (1990) Human Immunodeficiency Virus and Hepatitis B Virus Infections in Alcoholics. In D. Seminara et al. (Eds.), *Alcohol Immunomodulation, and AIDS.* pp. 67–73. New York: Alan R. Liss, Inc.

Johnson, R.W., Ostrow, D.G., & Joseph, J. (1990), Educational Strategies for Prevention of Sexual Transmission of HIV. In D.G. Ostrow (Ed.), *Behavioral Aspects of AIDS.* New York: Plenum Medical Book Company, pp. 43–73.

Kalichman, S.C., Kelly, J.A., Johnson, J.R., & Bulto, M. (1994). Factors Associated with risk for HIV Infection Among Chronic Mentally Ill Adults. *American Journal of Psychiatry. 151*, 221–227.

Kelly, J.A., Murphy, D.A., Bahr, G.R., Brasfield, T.L., Davis, D.R., Hauth, A.C., Morgan, M.G., Stevenson, L.Y., & Eilers, M.K. (1992). AIDS/HIV Risk Behavior Among the Chronic Mentally Ill. *American Journal of Psychiatry. 149*(7), 886–889.

Lauer-Listhaus, B., & Watterson, J. (1988). A Psychoeducational Group for HIV-Positive Patients on a Psychiatric Service. *Hospital and Community Psychiatry. 39*, 776–777.

Lee, H.K., Travin, S., & Blueston, H. (1992). Relationship Between HIV-1 Antibody Seropositivity and Alcohol/Nonintravenous Drug Abuse Among Psychiatric Inpatients: A Pilot Study. *American Journal of Addictions. 1*(1), 85–88.

Mahler, J.C., Perry, S., Yi, D., Sacks, M., & Dermatis, H. (1993). High, Undetected HIV Positive Rate on an Alcohol Rehabilitation Unit. *1993 New Research Program and Abstracts, 146th Annual Meeting of the American Psychiatric Association.* 207.

McDermott, B.E., Sautter, F.J., Winstead, D.K., & Quirk, T. (1994). Diagnosis, Health Beliefs, and Risk of HIV Infection in Psychiatric Patients. *Hospital and Community Psychiatry. 45*, 580–585.

Perry, S.W. (1990-a). AIDS and Psychiatry, In R. Michels (Ed), *Psychiatry*, Revised Edition, (p. 18), Philadelphia: J.B. Lippincott Company.

Perry, S.W. (1990-b). Organic Mental Disorders Caused by HIV: Update on Early Diagnosis and Treatment. *American Journal of Psychiatry. 147*(6), 696–710.

Sacks, M., Dermatis, H., Looser-Ott, S., & Perry, S. (1992). Seroprevalence of HIV and Risk Factors for AIDS in Psychiatric Inpatients. *Hospital and Community Psychiatry. 43*(7), 736–737.

Sacks, M.H., Perry, S., Graver, R., & Shindledecker, R. (1990). Self-Reported HIV-Related Risk Behaviors in Acute Psychiatric Inpatients: A Pilot Study. *Hospital and Community Psychiatry. 41*, 1253–1255.

Schleifer, S.J., & Keller, S.E. (1991). Psychoneuroimmunologic and Behavioral Issues in Populations at Risk for AIDS. *Psychiatric Medicine. 9*(3), 395–408.

Schmitt, F.A., Bigley, J.W., McKinnis, R., Logue, P.E., Evans, R.W., Drucker, J.L., and the AZT Collaborative Working Group (1988). Neuropsychological Outcome of Zidovudine (AZT) Treatment of Patients with AIDS and AIDS-Related Complex. *New England Journal of Medicine. 319*, 1573–1578.

Sladyk, K. (1990). Teaching Safe Sex Practices to Psychiatric Patients. *American Journal of Occupational Therapy, 44*, 284–286.

Stiffman, A.R., Dore, P., Earls, F., & Cunningham, R. (1992). The Influence of Mental Health Problems on AIDS-Related Risk Behaviors in Young Adults. *The Journal of Nervous and Mental Disease. 180*(5), 314–320.

Volavka, J., Convit, A, Czobor, P., Douyon, R., O'Donnell, J., & Ventura, F. (1991). HIV Seroprevalence and Risk Behaviors in Psychiatric Inpatients. *Psychiatry Research. 39*, 109–114.

11

Mental Disorders Secondary to Chronic Substance Abuse

JILL RACHBEISEL and DAVID MCDUFF

INTRODUCTION

Understanding and treating persons with dual diagnosis, including primary substance abusers with secondary mental disorders, necessitates a conceptual framework from which to work. Weiss and Collins (1992) organize the coexistence of mental illness and substance abuse into five categories:

1) The presence of an Axis I or Axis II disorder may act as a risk factor for substance abuse;

2) Psychiatric symptoms may develop in the course of chronic intoxication;

3) Psychiatric disorders may occur as a consequence of substance
    abuse and may persist after remission;

4) Substance abuse and psychiatric symptoms may be meaningful-
    ly linked over time; and

5) Substance abuse and psychiatric disorders may occur in the
    same individual but may be unrelated.

This chapter addresses the second and third categories: psychiatric illness that is a direct consequence of chronic substance abuse.

Differentiating substance-induced (ie., secondary) psychiatric illness from primary psychiatric illness is complex. Is the patient
demonstrating antisocial behavior to sustain an addiction, or does
primary sociopathy explain involvement in criminal activity and use
of illicit substances? Is the patient depressed because of chronic
exposure to cocaine or did a primary major depression trigger excessive use of cocaine in an effort to self medicate? These are common
clinical questions the answers to which are relevant for treatment
planning and outcome. Rounsaville and colleagues (1982-a, 1986)
demonstrate that the presence of a coexisting psychiatric diagnosis
in primary substance abusers generally predicts poorer treatment
outcome. Stoffelmayr, Benishek, Humphreys, Lee and Mavis (1989)
further point out that poor treatment outcome is related to
psychiatric symptom severity rather than the specific psychiatric
diagnosis.

Agreement on how to differentiate primary and secondary
psychiatric illness is lacking. Weiss and Collins (1992) summarize the
most common areas of disagreement. These include: 1) the timing of
psychiatric assessment, 2) the methods of collecting substance abuse
and psychiatric history, and 3) the sources of historical information.
Experts in the field disagree on how long an addict must be drug-free
before making another primary psychiatric diagnosis. Suggestions
range from two weeks (Dackis, Gold, Pattash, & Sweeney, 1986) to
three months (Schuckit, 1985). When considering how to collect the
information to make the diagnosis, many have opted to use structured clinical interviews such as the Diagnostic Interview Schedule
(Robins, Helzer, Craghan & Ratcliff, 1981) and the Structured Clinical
Interview for DSM (Spitzer, Williams & Gibbon, 1987). These
methods, however, have come under considerable criticism around

issues of reliability (Ford, Hilliard, Giesler, Lassen & Thomas, 1989). Since some patients may deny substance abuse or have inaccurate recall, collateral sources of information are recommended. Patients may also cite a secondary psychiatric illness as justification for substance abuse thereby confusing the chronology of events.

Several basic guidelines to help the clinician distinguish primary from secondary psychiatric disorders are listed below. These generalizations may vary slightly according to the specific drug of choice.

1) *Alcohol and Drug History*: To make a diagnosis of a substance-induced psychiatric disorder, the onset of the substance abuse must *predate* the onset of the psychiatric disorder. Therefore parallel time lines for recording the alcohol and drug history (including drugs used, frequency, and route of administration), psychiatric symptoms, and critical life events should be developed.

2) *Additional Sources*: All information should be substantiated by a second source that is considered reliable.

3) *Period of Abstinence*: The signs and symptoms of the suspected primary disorder must be clearly separate from those of acute intoxication or a withdrawal syndrome. A period of abstinence of at least four weeks is required to make this distinction.

4) *Previous Psychiatric Illness*: If an individual has had an episode of a psychiatric illness prior to drug use, episodes of psychiatric illness post-drugs must be considered primary unless the nature of the subsequent episodes differs significantly from that of the original episode (For example, the patient who suffered depressed mood as an adolescent from family conflict and now presents with a cocaine-induced depression).

5) *Family History*: Taking a careful family history of psychiatric illness is very important. A patient with more than one first degree relative with a primary psychiatric disorder is more likely to be suffering from a primary illness.

We will address the two most commonly observed severe and persistent psychiatric syndromes caused by substance abuse: major depression and psychosis. For both disorders we discuss diagnosis and psychopharmacologic treatments. We conclude with a general discussion of psychosocial interventions for persons with substance abuse and secondary chronic mental illness.

DEPRESSION

Diagnosis

Depressive symptoms are frequent among men and women with substance abuse. Chronic use of alcohol, opiates, and cocaine are the most common substances causing affective illness. Rounsaville, Anton, Carroll, Budde, Prusoff and Gawin (1991) identified the lifetime prevalence of major depression among opiate and cocaine abusers to be 54% and 30% respectively. Ross, Glaser and Germanson (1988) found a 22.6% lifetime prevalence for major depression and 13.4% lifetime prevalence for dysthymia in alcoholics.

The etiology of depression among substance abusers is multifactorial, and understanding the causes impacts greatly on the treatment approach. Jaffe and Ciraulo (1986) identify five common causes of depression in alcoholics: 1) toxic central nervous system and hepatic effects; 2) acute withdrawal syndrome; 3) social losses including jobs, friends, and family; 4) psychological awareness of the degree of functional impairment; and 5) personality disorders which impair the alcoholic's problem-solving and coping. These factors apply to other substances including opiates, cocaine, and sedative-hypnotics.

The types of depression seen with substance abuse are similar to the DSM-III primary depressive disorders except for reduced severity (mild to moderate rather than severe). Several studies demonstrate that depressive symptoms persist in abstinent substance abusers even though these patients do not always meet the DSM-III criteria (Pattenger, McKernon, Patrie, Weissman, Ruben, & Newberry, 1978). Jaffe and Ciraulo (1986) found the same results in a study of alcoholics in a Veteran population. Rounsaville, Weissman, Kleber and Wilber (1982-b) studied opiate addicts and found that depressive syndromes were common and were characterized by comparatively mild symptomatology. The symptoms that most commonly linger are dysphoria and low self-esteem.

Assessing for the presence of a depressive disorder should be done carefully and over a time span that permits the clinician to distinguish those symptoms which are associated with acute intoxication or a withdrawal syndrome from those which persist well into abstinence. In most cases the depressive symptoms will be most severe following immediate cessation of the substance and improve with abstinence. This is typically the case with alcohol and opiate abuse. The alcoholic who presents with depressive symptoms can often have complete resolution of the symptoms within one to two weeks (Schuckit, 1986; Jaffe & Ciraulo, 1986). Depressions associated with opiate dependence also show significant improvement with abstinence and involvement in a treatment program shortly after entry and most are completely resolved after six months (Rounsaville et al., 1982-a).

Rawson, Obet and McCann (1991) describe the following sequence after cession of cocaine use: 1) withdrawal stage: the ("coke crash"), which is usually identified as Days 0–15 and characterized by severe but short lived depression; 2) "honeymoon" stage: (approximately Days 16–45) during which time the patient experiences improved mood, energy and optimism, and decreased craving; 3) "wall" stage: (Days 46–120) which is viewed as a major obstacle in the cocaine recovery process. During the wall phase, low energy, anhedonia, irritability, difficulty concentrating, poor libido and insomnia return. Feelings of hopelessness intensify and relapse vulnerability is at an all time high.

Treatment

The clinician must emphasize the primary importance of treating the substance abuse when depression is identified as a secondary problem. Depressive symptoms can be viewed as barriers to recovery or relapse triggers and can be managed as an aspect of the recovery program. The psychosocial aspects of treatment will be discussed in a later section. However, the physician often struggles with the use of pharmacologic interventions early in the course of treatment. There are several factors to be considered when addressing this question:

1) *Severity of Symptoms*: Suicide, often associated with depression, is a serious concern. Fifteen to twenty-five percent of suicides are committed by alcoholics and 5–27% of all deaths in alcoholics are due to suicide as compared to 1% in the general population (Jaffe and Ciraulo, 1986). However, there are other factors that contribute to the incidence of suicide in addition to depression including intoxication, disinhibition, and social losses (Murphy, Armstrong & Hermele, 1979). A patient with persistent suicidal thinking, hopelessness, and despair well into the period of abstinence should be considered for a trial of medication. Individuals who have already made a serious suicide attempt, particularly if they were not in a state of

intoxication at the time, are at higher risk and should be considered for medication.

2) *Level of Functioning*: The patient's level of functioning after an adequate period of abstinence must be monitored. If the depression has continued to impair the individual's occupational, interpersonal, or social functioning well below what would be expected *for that person*, medication may be appropriate.

3) *Record of Relapse*: If the depressive symptoms are interfering with recovery and are thought to be fueling relapse, pharmacotherapy may be an option. A substance abuser who has multiple relapses in a relatively short period of time and continues to complain of depression may be a candidate for medication.

There are several difficult issues that surface when using medication with depressed substance abusers. The first is the increased risk of suicide when administering antidepressants in the presence of active substance use. The second is the ideological conflict that occurs from using mood-altering medications in recovering patients, (ie: the act of "taking a pill to feel better" may defeat the very goal of recovery). Third, the push for short hospital stays often leaves the psychiatrist with inadequate time to fully assess the depression. A seven to ten day hospital stay is often too short to ascertain whether the patient needs medication or remains at risk for relapse or suicide. Shortened stays frequently lead the physician to medicate prematurely.

To summarize, most secondary depressive syndromes related to substance abuse are milder forms of the primary disorders and tend to improve and resolve with abstinence and time. Pharmacologic intervention is indicated, however, when the depressive symptoms persist and result in a continued suicide risk, impair functioning or cause repeated relapses.

Controlled studies evaluating drug effectiveness in these persons are inconsistent and inadequate. Nevertheless, some discussion of the different medications available is warranted. The tricyclic antidepressants (TCA's) are appropriate for alcoholics who have been sober for at least four weeks but remain depressed. The potential lethality of the combination of alcohol and the TCA's must be considered, and the compliance and reliability of the patient assessed. Frequent office visits and limited supplies of medications may provide a safe approach for some patients. Monoamine oxidase inhibitors (MAOI) are difficult to use since they require careful dietary restrictions and have a potential for liver toxicity. In a population that is often impulsive this class of medication is not practical. Lithium has been investigated for relapse prevention but has not been found to be effective in the treatment of an alcoholic depression. The serotonin re-uptake inhibitors, (e.g., fluoxetine, paroxetine and sertraline) may be the safest class of medications for use in this population. Overdose potential is much lower. Although they have not been studied specifically in this population, they have been found to be equally effective for primary depression when compared to the TCA's. The above approach is applicable to the opiate addict as well.

The treatment of cocaine addiction with antidepressants has received much research attention. Kosten et al. (1992) completed a six month follow-up study on patients who had participated in a desipramine trial. There were significantly decreased episodes of depression in the treated group compared to the placebo group and a much higher rate of abstinence. Meta-analysis conducted with nine separate studies assessing the efficacy of desipramine treatment in cocaine addicts also showed that there was increased abstinence in addicts who remained on medication (Levin & Lehman, 1991). This suggests that the use of desipramine is a reasonable first choice in this group.

PSYCHOTIC DISORDERS

Diagnosis

Secondary psychotic disorders have been identified in relation to a wide variety of addictive substances including alcohol, cocaine, marijuana, and benzodiazepines. Many designer drugs also have an associated psychotic syndrome. The mescaline analogs (ecstasy, crystal ice), arylhexylamines (phencyclidine), and crack cocaine are included in this group (Beebe & Walley, 1991). Psychotic episodes can be divided into two subtypes: 1) acute psychosis associated with intoxication or a withdrawal syndrome; and 2) chronic residual psychosis as a result of chronic substance abuse.

Drugs commonly found to have an associated acute psychotic component in the intoxicated state include phencyclidine (PCP), crack cocaine, and the hallucinogens. PCP, also referred to as "angel dust" or "dust," is most commonly smoked but can be ingested or snorted with cocaine and has an onset of action within one minute of inhalation or one hour of ingestion. It is known to inhibit presynaptic uptake of norepinephrine, dopamine, and serotonin. In low doses, euphoria and depersonalization are experienced. At higher doses, the user becomes combative, paranoid, and unpredictable. Acute PCP toxicity produces acute psychosis with delusional thinking and auditory hallucinations. Cocaine can also produce a state of arousal and hypervigilence that can present as suspiciousness and progress to paranoia or more severely as a paranoid psychosis. Acute toxicity may result in visual hallucinations referred to as "snow lights" or tactile hallucinations commonly referred to as "cocaine bugs" (Beebe & Walley, 1991). The hallucinogens such as LSD are also associated with a psychotic episode characterized by depersonalization, delusional thinking and paranoid ideation. Bizarre experiences are often reported such as synesthesia (i.e., seeing smells and hearing colors). Touch is magnified and time is markedly distorted. Marijuana intoxication can also precipitate a psychotic state. There is much controversy, however, as to whether this is a true secondary illness, "cannabis psychosis," or a presentation of an underlying primary disorder. In some susceptible people a toxic psychosis directly caused by the marijuana has been described. This effect resolves as the drug is metabolized. The syndrome includes restlessness, confusion, bewilderment, fear, illusions, and hallucinations (Grinspoon & Bakalor, 1992).

States of withdrawal which induce psychotic symptoms are seen with alcohol and sedative-hypnotics. The well described alcohol withdrawal syndrome (delirium tremens) is characterized by extreme agitation and visual and tactile hallucinations generally remitting hours to days after onset. Untreated sedative-hypnotic withdrawal can lead to a similar delirious state of disorientation, extreme anxiety and hallucinations, both visual and auditory.

Chronic psychotic syndromes secondary to drug abuse are seen with alcoholism and some of the designer drugs, specifically 3,4-methylenedioxymethamphetamine (ecstasy or MDMA). Alcohol causes several separate psychotic syndromes which are due to the direct effects of the alcohol on the central nervous system and to vitamin deficiencies. Alcoholic hallucinosis is a syndrome usually associated with cessation of drinking and is time-limited. There are, however, individuals with a history of years of severe drinking who develop hallucinations which do not remit even with prolonged abstinence. Wernicke-Korsakov psychosis is another illness which is a direct result of severe vitamin B_1 (thiamine) deficiency. Amnestic periods and severe short term memory loss accompanied by confabulation are present. There can also be co-existing delirium, misrecognition of others and misperception of situations. Alcohol induced hypomagnesemia can lead to increased irritability and suspiciousness. This condition can progress to paranoid delusions (Giannini & Collins, 1992). Ecstasy or MDMA is a mescaline analog which renders the user euphoric and with a heightened sense of self esteem. Chronic use of ecstasy can result in a paranoid psychotic state that is clinically identical to schizophrenia. This condition can resolve after a prolonged state of abstinence.

Treatment

Pharmacological treatment of secondary psychosis falls into two basic approaches similar to the classifications: 1) a brief course of treatment for the acute episodes of psychosis, and 2) long-term management of the chronic conditions. In the psychotic states of acute cocaine, PCP, and LSD intoxication, supportive treatments are optimal. Providing a safe, non-threatening, quiet environment with verbal reassurance is often most effective. Cocaine intoxication is self-limiting and detoxification can take less than 24 hours. Benzodiazepines should be avoided, such as for the management of extreme anxiety that can accompany cocaine withdrawal, because they can mask other significant complications that require medical interventions (e.g., hypertensive crisis or cardiac arrhythmias). The exception is the management of seizures which rarely accompany cocaine withdrawal and are effectively treated with diazepam.

PCP intoxication and withdrawal, often characterized by violence and hyperactivity, are best managed with supportive interventions and minimal stimulation. Benzodiazepines are useful for control of severe agitation. Antipsychotic medications should be avoided for the first 24 hours of acute intoxication since the anticholinergic side effects enhance the toxic effects of PCP. However, when psychosis persists, haloperidol is the drug of choice in managing the violent, psychotic PCP-intoxicated patient, and low dosing (5 mg.) on an as needed basis is usually all that is required. These same guidelines should be applied to LSD intoxication.

In the case of the withdrawal syndromes from alcohol or sedative-hypnotics, a steady, smooth, and slow detoxification with a long-acting benzodiazepine is the most effective management. If the patient is appropriately detoxified, a severe psychotic event will be avoided. In the event of persistent hallucinations, such as in alcoholic hallucinosis, a low dose antipsychotic is effective. Once the acute intoxication or withdrawal syndrome is resolved, there is no need to continue maintenance medications. The patient should be discharged and maintained drug free.

In the chronic psychotic states of alcoholism, the specific etiology must be identified. In the case of Wernicke-Korsakov psychosis, thiamine replacement must be emergently administered intramuscularly or intravenously on the first day and orally on a daily basis for the next 6–12 months. About half of the patients will demonstrate some recovery over time after 5 years. One fourth will show no improvement. If magnesium deficiency is identified, intramuscular magnesium sulfate should be given daily to titrate serum levels to normal. Antipsychotic medications are indicated and effective in the management of the irreversible hallucinations and delusions. Low doses of high potency antipsychotic are preferable.

GENERAL TREATMENT ISSUES

The most important aspect of the treatment of any mental disorder secondary to substance abuse is the treatment of addiction. This treatment consists of working towards abstinence from all mood altering drugs, drug education, individual therapy, group therapy, and involvement in self-help groups. Below is a brief comment on each of these aspects.

Abstinence is the ideal goal that a substance abuser must achieve in order to effectively treat the resultant psychiatric illness. It is unrealistic, however, to expect individuals to achieve this goals in a single step, particularly if they are in the pre-treatment phase of recovery. This phase is the point at which persons have not actually entered active treatment and are often in a state of denial about their addiction and the impact that substance use has on their mental illness. A more effective approach is a slow, progressive beginning with simple open communication about what drugs are used. In this way the individual can more easily engage in treatment and is less likely to drop out.

Drug education includes information about the physiological, psychological and social impacts that drug and alcohol use have on a person and enables a better understanding of the development of symptoms. Time spent on the interplay of addiction and mental illness as well as a review of the similarities between mental illness and addiction helps abusers to reorganize their understanding of their behavior and emotional response to situations.

Brief, recovery-oriented psychotherapy is used to engage relapse-prone patients with substance abuse and to diminish psychiatric symptoms which can serve as recovery barriers. It has been shown in a preliminary study that this form of therapy can lead to an increased retention in treatment (McDuff & Slounias, 1992). Therapy is time-limited, from 4 to 8 sessions, and focuses only on issues related to relapse of substance abuse. Six issues commonly dealt with are reviewed below.

1) The therapeutic focus can include negative affective states (anger, depression, anxiety, emptiness, guilt) where work centralizes around understanding how emotion relates to substance use. Keeping a symptom diary and relating this to actual daily use of drugs and alcohol is useful in helping the patient make the connections and then moving on in therapy to learning new coping mechanisms.

2) Traumatic events are often a therapeutic focus since many substance abusers have been victims of rape, incest, or assault. As a result of these violent crimes, they have assumed the role of "helpless, passive victim" and this passivity has a negative impact on their ability to take an active role in their recovery. The therapy focuses on reframing the individual's response to the violent event as acceptable within the framework that it occurred, thereby releasing patients from the intense feelings of guilt and shame and enabling them to enter recovery in an active frame of mind.

3) Character pathology or individuals' interpersonal styles often bring them to therapy because of their difficulty in getting along with other patients or staff in treatment programs. The work focuses on having patients identify ways their behavior interferes with the program. Common issues identified include impulsivity, inability to trust others, acting out, and antisocial behavior. Exploring alternative coping strategies while in active treatment can enhance quality and quantity of time spent in recovery.

4) Unresolved grief ia another common focus. Working through the loss of a loved one in therapy can also be a model for addicts to

work through the process of giving up addictive life style on which they have come to depend.

5) Developmental arrest often becomes a therapeutic focus when abusers report they are stuck at an earlier phase of life and feel left behind. These patients acknowledge a need to grow up but are at a loss at how to do it. Therapy focuses on the identification of age appropriate behaviors in others and then applying them during treatment to themselves.

6) Persistent denial as the therapeutic focus occurs when the abuser is not able to engage in treatment despite repeated attempts. The therapist often takes a non-confrontational approach in order to minimize defensiveness and organizes the therapy around examining the patient's drinking style and patterns, looking for evidence of loss of control, use despite of consequences, or compulsiveness. Asking the patient what else would have to change in order to stop an addiction is an alternative to confrontation that then minimizes their resistance.

Group therapy and self-help groups together provide the recovering addict with an adequate support network. Validation of feelings, recognition of difficulties in recovery, and positive feedback to enhance self-esteem are outcomes of consistent groupwork in recovery.

CONCLUSION

Careful history taking, assessment of psychiatric signs and symptoms in relation to intoxication and withdrawal, and an adequate period of abstinence are essential to the diagnosis of a secondary chronic mental disorder. Concurrent treatment of the mental illness and addiction is necessary since treatment of either in isolation is bound to fail. Extreme caution should be exercised when selecting psychotropic medications, avoiding those with high addictive potential. Most importantly, abstinence must be the eventual and ultimate goal thereby assisting with the resolution of the psychiatric symptoms and prevention of further episodes.

REFERENCES

Beebe, D. K., & Walley, E.: (1991). Substance abuse: The designer drugs. *American Family Physician, 43,* 1689–1698.

Dackis, C. A., Gold, M. S., Pattash, A. L. C., & Sweeney, E. R. (1986). Evaluating depression in alcoholics. *Psychiatry Research, 17,* 105–109.

Ford, J., Hilliard, J. R., Giesler, L. J., Lassen, K. L., & Thomas, H. (1989). Substance abuse/mental illness: Diagnostic issues. *American Journal of Drug and Alcohol Abuse. 15,* 297–307.

Giannini, A. J., & Collins, G. B. (1992) Substance abuse and thought disorders. In *Dual Diagnosis in Substance Abuse.* (pp. 57–93) New York: Marcel Dekker, Inc.

Grinspoon, L., & Bakalor, J. B. (1992). Marijuana substance abuse. In Lowinson, J., Ruiz, P., & Millman, R. B. (Eds.), *Substance Abuse: A Comprehensive Textbook* (pp. 236–246), Baltimore: Williams & Wilkens.

Jaffe, J. H., & Ciraulo, D. A. (1986). Alcoholism and depression. In R. E. Meyer (Ed.), *Psychopathology and Addictive Disorders* (pp. 293–320), New York: Guilford Press.

Kosten, T. R., Gawin, F. H., Kosten, T. A., Morgan, C., Rounsaville, B. J., Schottenfeld, R., & Kleber, H.D. (1992). Six-month follow-up of short-term pharmacotherapy for cocaine dependence. *American Journal of Addictions. 1,* 40–49.

Levin, F. R., & Lehman, A. F. (1991). Meta-analysis of desipramine as an adjunct in the treatment of cocaine addiction. *Journal of Clinical Psychopharmacology, 11*(6), 374–378.

McDuff, D. R., & Solounias, B. L. (1992). The use of brief psychotherapy with substance abusers in early recovery. *Journal of Psychotherapy Practice and Research, 1*(2), 163–170.

Murphy, G. E., Armstrong, J. W., & Hermele, S. L. (1979). Suicide and alcoholism. *Archives of General Psychiatry, 36,* 65–69.

Pattenger, M., McKernon, J., Patrie, L. E., Weissman, M. M., Ruben, H. L., & Newberry, P. (1978). The frequency and persistence of depressive symptoms in the alcohol abuser. *Journal of Nervous and Mental Disorders, 166,* 562–570.

Pettinati, H. M., Sugerman, A. A., & Mauer H. S. (1982). Four year MMPI changes in abstinent and drinking alcoholics. *Alcoholism: Clinical and Experimental Research, 199,* 482–487.

Rawson, R. A., Obert, J. L., & McCann, M. J. (1991). Cocaine: Recovery issues. *Addiction and Recovery, 11,* 29–33.

Robins, L. N., Helzer, J. E., Croughan, J., & Ratcliff, K. S. (1981). National Institute of Mental Health diagnostic interview schedule. *Archives of General Psychiatry, 38*, 81–389.

Ross, H. E., Glaser, F. B., & Germanson, T. (1988). The prevalence of psychiatric disorders in patients with alcohol and other drug problems. *Archives of General Psychiatry, 45*, 1023–1031.

Rounsaville, B. J., Anton, S. F., Carroll, K., Budde, D., Prusoff, B. A., & Gawin, F. (1991). Psychiatric diagnosis of treatment-seeking cocaine abusers. *Archives of General Psychiatry, 48*, 43–51.

Rounsaville, B. J., Kosten, T. R., Weissman, M. M., & Kleber, H. (1986) Prognostic significance of psychopathology in treated opiate addicts. *Archives of General Psychiatry, 43*, 739–745.

Rounsaville, B. J., Weissman, M. M., Crits-Christoph, K., Wilber, C., & Kleber, H. (1982-a). Diagnosis and symptoms of depression in opiate addicts. *Archives of General Psychiatry, 39*, 151–156.

Rounsaville, B. J., Weissman, M. M., Kleber, H., & Wilber, C. (1982-b). Heterogeneity of psychiatric diagnosis in treated opiate addicts. *Archives of General Psychiatry, 39*, 161–166.

Schuckit, M. A. (1985). The clinical implications of primary diagnostic groups among alcoholics. *Archives of General Psychiatry, 42*, 1043–1049.

Schuckit, M. A. (1986). Genetic and clinical implications of alcoholism and affected disorder. *American Journal of Psychiatry, 143*, 140–147.

Spitzer, R. L., Williams, J. B. W., & Gibbon, M. A. (1987). Structured clinical interview for DSM III-R. Biometrics Research Department, New York State Psychiatric Institute, New York.

Stoffelmayr, B. E., Benishek, L. A., Humphreys, K., Lee, J. A., & Mavis, B. E. (1989). Substance abuse prognosis with an additional psychiatric diagnosis: Understanding the relationship. *Journal of Psychoactive Drugs, 21*(2), 145–152.

Weiss, R. D., & Collins, D. A. (1992). Substance abuse and psychiatric illness: The dually diagnosed patient. *American Journal of Addictions, 1*, 93–99.

Section III:

Social System Issues

12

The Family and the Dually Diagnosed Patient

KATHLEEN SCIACCA and AGNES B. HATFIELD

Families of patients with dual disorders experience the disruptions due to addictive disorders in addition to the stressors of coping with a serious mental illness. Although many studies (Hatfield, 1987-a; Lefley, 1987; Marsh, 1992) have shown that families of mentally ill relatives report enormous amounts of stress due to mental illness, there are few studies that have assessed the added burden due to substance abuse problems. One study (Kashner et.al., 1991) reported that substance abuse contributes to family conflict, erodes social support, and generates high levels of expressed emotion, thus disturbing the vitally needed caregiving network. Therefore, it is important to provide services for families.

The National Alliance for the Mentally Ill (NAMI) is an advocacy group that began from grass roots movements of families with mentally ill relatives in the 1970's and has since grown to over 1,000 local chapters (Grosser & Vine, 1991). The "family movement" has a strong influence on research and treatment of individuals with severe and persistent mental illness (U.S. News and World Report, 1989). However, many family members accept a mental health system and a substance abuse system that do not address their relative's addictive disorders.

NAMI recently conducted a national survey of family perspectives on meeting the needs of people with mental illness (Steinwachs, Kasper, & Skinner, 1992) and found that 18 per cent of the respondents indicated that getting drunk or using drugs occurred in their families. Of these families, 62 per cent considered this to be a serious problem. It is important to note that the 18 per cent rate of substance abuse reported in the NAMI study is much lower than most other studies report as indicated in Chapter 2 of this volume. The lower rate reported in the NAMI study may be explained in one of several ways. Members of NAMI are not fully representative of all families with mentally ill relatives. It is possible that there is less substance abuse in their relatives. It is equally possible that families believe mental illness is the primary source of disturbance and overlook the substance abuse. Some families may not be able to distinguish problems due to mental illness from those due to substance abuse. Still others may deny the problem out of shame, guilt or embarrassment.

Dually diagnosed patients have been characterized as systems misfits with poor outcome, more relapses, more acting out behavior, and more likelihood of being homeless (Minkoff and Drake, 1991). Despite the serious consequences of drug and alcohol abuse in persons with mental illness, the family movement has not attained the same degree of knowledge about addictive disorders as they have about mental illness. Understanding mental illness as a disease that is not caused by families was necessary to establish successful advocacy for persons with mental illness. The same advocacy and education are essential to help those who are dually diagnosed through a clear understanding of the addictive disorders. Families of dually diagnosed persons continue to experience frustration resulting from a service delivery system that does not meet their needs or the needs of their relatives.

The purpose of this chapter is to discuss some of the issues and problems associated with helping families who have dually diagnosed members, and to outline a model program, "MICAA-NON," for families of the dually diagnosed. (MICAA stands for Mental Illness Chemical Abuse and Addiction). We will begin by clarifying some of the areas that affect the delivery of services. Next we will report on our family survey, the Maryland study, which provides a family perspective of the issues. This will be followed by an outline of a pioneer program and some assessment considerations.

ISSUES THAT IMPEDE SERVICES FOR DUALLY DIAGNOSED PERSONS AND THEIR FAMILIES

Both families and providers encounter difficulties in accessing comprehensive services for dually diagnosed persons. These difficulties include: 1) Bureaucracies divided according to individual categories of disorders with segregated admissions criteria, treatment programs, services, and reimbursement; 2) Providers who are educated and trained to deliver services for single disorders only (Ridgely, Goldman & Willenbring, 1990); and, 3) Treatment approaches across disorders that are incompatible and differ in method and philosophy (Sciacca, 1991).

As discussed in Chapter 5, a significant issue is the contrasting treatment methods used by providers in the different fields. Traditional treatment methods for drug addiction and alcoholism are usually intense and confrontational. They are designed to break down the patient's denial or resistance of his or her addictive disorder. Admissions criteria to substance abuse programs usually require abstinence from all illicit substances. Potential patients are expected to be aware of the problems caused by substance abuse, and motivated to receive treatment. In some programs the use of medication is unacceptable. This automatically excludes people who take prescribed medication for their symptoms of mental illness. In contrast, treatment methods used for serious mental illness are supportive, benign and non-threatening. They are designed to maintain the patient's often fragile defenses. Criteria for admission into mental health services rarely require that patients are aware of their substance abuse problems and motivated to accept substance abuse treatment. Patients entering the mental health system are generally not seeking treatment for their substance abuse problems and, while actively abusing drugs and alcohol, deny such use, a finding supported by the study of Maryland families described below (see Table 12.1).

These differences perpetuate the gaps in services and often exclude dually diagnosed persons from existing services. Traditional substance abuse services may not accept patients who have a serious mental illness either because they do not meet the readiness criteria, or because they are not prepared to provide services for symptoms of mental illness. If accepted into a substance abuse program that is not modified, dually diagnosed patients may experience difficulty when participating in an intense, confrontational program. Traditionally, the mental health system attempts to exclude dually diagnosed patients on the basis of substance abuse at the time of admission. For patients within the system, services are interrupted or terminated for violations of rules regarding addictive behaviors. Families who do not understand the addictions as disorders will accept these determinations. Without knowledge of the necessity of professional treatment, family members are not likely to perceive their relative's entitlement to addiction treatment. The result is frustration and hardship for families who have the burden of caring for a relative who does not receive the benefits of professional help, or the pain and fear involved when a family can no longer provide primary care. In such cases, their dually diagnosed relative loses the support of both the family and the service systems. Community residences and other alternative living programs for mentally ill persons exclude dually diagnosed patients by using criteria to screen out substance abusers. These program options are rarely accessible alternatives.

Working with patients who deny substance abuse, who are unmotivated for substance abuse treatment, and are unable to tolerate intense confrontation, requires a new model of treatment. Sciacca developed a "non-confrontational" approach to the engagement and treatment of persons who are dually diagnosed. The treatment model first developed by Sciacca in 1984 (Sciacca, 1987-a) is based upon non-judgmental acceptance of all symptoms and experiences related to both mental illness and substance abuse. The phase by phase interventions from "denial" to "abstinence" (Sciacca, 1991) begin by assessing the patient's readiness to engage in treatment (Sciacca, 1990). Readiness levels are accepted as starting points for treatment, rather than points for elimination.

These programs (MICAA treatment groups) are implemented as components of existing mental health, or substance abuse programs, "Integrated Treatment." They have been adapted to a wide variety of services including short- and long-term inpatient units, acute care services, outpatient clinics, day treatment programs, continuing care programs, case management services, community residences, shelters, and clubhouse models of service (Sciacca, 1987-b).

A FAMILY PERSPECTIVE ON DUAL DIAGNOSIS: THE MARYLAND STUDY

With little or no data available on how families view the problem of substance abuse and mental illness, we asked families in the Maryland Alliance for the Mentally Ill who had such a problem to complete a brief survey. While the number of usable responses was limited to 22, we report on these responses along with published information on the subject in order to identify family problems and needs. The majority of dually diagnosed individuals identified in this study were young men with a long history of drug and/or alcohol abuse which preceded the onset of their mental illness.

Consequences of Substance Abuse

Families in the Maryland study were asked to identify the behavior problems and increased symptomatology they believed were due to substance use as summarized in Table 12.1. It is important in interpreting this table to recognize that some families noted that it was hard to separate problems due to substance abuse from those due to mental illness.

A majority of families reported that denial (77%) and money problems (77%) were troublesome to them. Well over half (59%) indicated that legal difficulties, blaming others, and being argumentative were very troublesome behaviors and nearly as many (55%) were concerned about decline in health and loss of jobs. When asked which problems were the **most** troublesome, the most common response was denial of the problem and decline in health. These then are the areas in which families need help from providers.

Respondents said that rehospitalization was required for 88% of their relatives and that 77% had acute symptoms of mental illness evoked by their alcohol or drug use. The symptoms most often mentioned were: depression (59%); suicidal ideation (59%); voices (55%); violence (36%); visual hallucinations (23%), and; blackouts (23%).

Reasons for Substance Abuse Problems

Although it may not be possible to know the etiology of substance abuse in a reliable way, it is important to know what families believe

Table 12.1. Behavioral Problems Due to
Substance Abuse ($N = 22$)

Problem	Percent with problem
Denial of problem*	77%
Money problems	77%
Legal difficulty	59%
Blaming others	59%
Argumentativeness	59%
Decline in health*	55%
Loss of job	55%
Lying	45%
Loss of housing	41%
Violence	41%
Accidents	41%
Manipulating	41%
Stealing	23%
Sexual misconduct	4%

*Labeled by respondents as most troublesome.

because it may influence the way they respond to their relative's problem. Families in the Maryland study were asked to check as many reasons for substance abuse as they believe applied to their relative (Table 12.2).

It is interesting to note that most families (68%) felt that self-medication is one of the reasons for their relative's reliance on alcohol and/or drug use. Just over half (55%) viewed substance abuse as a disease that needs treatment and 55 per cent felt that one explanation lies in an underlying psychological problem. Boredom and the search for a social life were given as further reasons. Only one respondent felt that substance abuse was evidence of weak character.

Treatments Used and Their Effectiveness

An important objective of the Maryland study was to determine families' perceptions of what treatments for substance abuse were

Table 12.2. Families' Perceptions of Reasons for
Substance Abuse ($N = 22$)

Reasons for abuse	Percent of families reporting
Attempts at self medication	68%
A disease that needs treatment	55%
Response to psychological problems	55%
Fills time and overcomes boredom	32%
Forms the basis of a social life	27%
Has weak character	5%

available to their dually diagnosed relatives and how well these treatments were working. Sixty-eight percent of patients had ever been treated for substance abuse disorders and the treatments used were variable. Of note, nearly one third of patients had no treatment. Table 12.3 shows the most frequently used services in the Maryland study and how families rated their effectiveness.

Family members named group therapy and Alcoholics and Anonymous/Narcotics Anonymous (A.A./N.A.) as the most common services utilized. While both were rated as fair or good in effectiveness, A.A./N.A was felt to be superior. Although used less often (36%), individual therapy was seen as having equal effectiveness to group therapy. Detoxification was rated as effective, but, as one respondent noted, it was only of temporary value.

What is of most interest for the purposes of this chapter was that while only 36 per cent of families were involved in the treatment of their relative, all of them rated the effectiveness of this involvement as fair or good. This supports the recommendations of a number of authorities (Sciacca, 1991; Evans & Sullivan, 1990) that families should receive special services or be included in the treatment.

Special Services Needed

Since families are in a position to observe their relatives over time and to note their reactions to various treatments, their perceptions about

Table 12.3. Treatments Used and Their Effectiveness ($N = 22$)

Treatment	Percent using	Effectiveness	
		Poor	Fair/Good
Group therapy	50%	36%	64%
A.A/N.A	50%	9%	91%
Hospitalization	41%	33%	67%
Individual therapy	36%	38%	62%
Detoxification	36%	13%	87%
Family Involvement	36%	0	100%

the special services needed are especially important. Table 12.4 shows the responses of the Maryland families to questions about service needs.

Families felt that special outpatient services (82%) were much more needed than inpatient services (39%). Over half of the group felt that special crisis intervention, special self-help groups, and special residences need to be available. Of interest to us was the need expressed for special family support groups (64%).

OBSTACLES TO PROVIDING SERVICES FOR FAMILIES OF DUALLY DIAGNOSED PERSONS

Services for families of dually diagnosed persons are an important complement to the treatment process. Prior to, and apart from our Maryland study, numerous families reported devastating experiences stemming from their efforts to access services, and from the stressors of caring for a dually diagnosed relative (Sciacca, 1989).

Traditional twelve step programs for family members of alcoholics, Al-Anon, often do not meet the needs of a family whose relative also has a mental illness. Concepts such as "hitting bottom" (Al-Anon, 1984) are not easily acceptable to families of dually diagnosed people. For a dually diagnosed person, hitting bottom may result in decompensation into acute symptoms, deterioration of functioning, loss of supports, and hospitalization. Families also fear the potential dangers involved in "putting their relative out on the

Table 12.4. Families' Perceptions of Special Services
Needed for Dually Diagnosed Individuals

Special services needed	Percent of families
Special outpatient treatment programs	82%
More trained providers in dual diagnosis	68%
Special family support groups	64%
Appropriate crisis intervention	59%
Special self-help groups	59%
Special residences	50%
Inpatient treatment	39%

street," which may be construed as a necessary action for families of addicted individuals. Programs such as Al-Anon are not comprehensive, and do not address mental illness or the interactions of mental illness and substance disorders.

When traditional supports and services are not sufficient, families of dually diagnosed persons rely upon the mental health system for support. Presently, there are few services within that system to address their needs. Alliance for the Mentally Ill (AMI) local chapters include families of dually diagnosed persons, but they usually constitute a less cohesive subgroup. As a result, many chapters do not provide the additional specialized supports. At the national and several statewide levels, NAMI attempts to address the issues of the family with dually diagnosed members (Hatfield, 1992). This includes efforts to educate all of the membership.

MICAA-NON: AN EDUCATION AND SUPPORT FOR FAMILIES

Without the development of specialized services for dually diagnosed patients there is virtually no consideration given to the special needs of their families. As an outgrowth of the attention given to the treatment needs of the patients under MICAA programs, the serious needs of their family members came to fore. As a model family program was developed, it paralleled the intervention process adapted to dually diagnosed patients in several important ways.

Initially, a patient in denial is engaged to participate in an educational group where he or she may learn about substance disorders (Sciacca, 1991). Providers trained to work with patients at this phase create a non-threatening environment and employ interventions that foster trust among the leader and the group members. When patients recognize that it is safe to discuss one's own use of substances, progress has been made along the continuum. They move from denial of substance use, to openly discussing their use of substance in a supportive environment.

Interventions necessary to assist the client to the next step of readiness or recovery are continually employed. For example, a patient who has reached the point of readiness to discuss his or her substance use may deny any negative consequences. Through concerned exploration and education about the effects of substance a-buse, the patient is assisted along the continuum to recognize specific problems and interactions of substance abuse with mental illness. This process continues until abstinence, the goal, is achieved. Specific education about mental illness and substance abuse is essential to this treatment process (Sciacca, 1991).

MICAA-NON began in 1987 (Sciacca, 1989) in an effort to educate families about mental illness, drug addiction and alcoholism. It began with presentations at local AMI chapters. Chapter presidents forewarned that many members were resistent toward openly discussing substance abuse issues. As a result, educational meetings rather than support groups were offered as a follow-up to presentations. The engagement process used with dually diagnosed patients was applied here. Participants need not disclose information about their dually diagnosed relative. Interest in learning about the addictive disorders and their interactions with mental illness was the only prerequisite.

The first MICAA-NON meetings included some families who were not ready to discuss their relative's substance abuse, while other families did so openly. Family members had tales of isolation, disrupted lives, and uncertainty as to where to go for help. They clearly lacked a forum to discuss these problems. Families reported having their input ignored while their relative received treatment that did not account for the substance abuse problem. Similar reports were given by families who attended presentations at statewide AMI

and national NAMI conferences. Frequently, these were initial dis-
closures of experiences that had long been harbored in silence. Em-
pirically, this confirmed the extent of the need for education and
support for families of dually diagnosed people.

MICAA-NON Program Outline

MICAA-NON groups require the leadership of an informed provider
who can assist families to acquire services and develop networks from
limited resources. When developing treatment programs for dually
diagnosed persons, some agencies extend their services to include a
MICAA-NON program. Staff members in training at such agencies
learn to lead family meetings under supervision (Sciacca, 1991).
Through educating and learning from families, they gain insight into
the broader network and experiences of their dually diagnosed
patients. They understand the family and the patient as a system and
learn new ways to work together. As the plight of the family unfolds,
providers begin to let go of outworn theories of families as causal to
mental illness (Lefley, 1987-a). Instead, they recognize the support
families provide, often under extremely adverse conditions.

MICAA-NON groups have not been developed for profit. When
a group begins it is open to all families throughout the community.
Participants need not have a patient in treatment at the sponsoring
agency. Many families who do attend have the presenting problem
of a relative who either refuses or is unable to access appropriate
treatment.

Groups include multiple families and do not usually include the
patient. Meetings of three to twelve participants are usually held in
the evening on a weekly, bi-monthly or monthly basis as decided by
members. They last approximately one and one-half to two hours.
MICAA-NON groups need to be ongoing and should continue for
as long as the resources (leader, space, sponsoring agency) are available.

Outreach is very important to the formation of groups and sustaining membership. A presentation at a local AMI chapter or other
family programs begin with a general overview of the disease concepts of mental illness, drug addiction and alcoholism. Participants
are given the opportunity to sign up to attend additional educational
meetings. They are notified of the details of each meeting in writing
and by telephone the day of the meeting. Flyers and notices are

strategically sent to reach as many agencies and family members as possible. Notices are placed in local newsletters.New members may join at any time. Participants are encouraged to invite other families, as well as additional members of their own family.

MICAA-NON Program Content

The content of the meetings includes both support and education. Following introductions, participants share in an open discussion. Usually, at least one member will discuss a personal issue. The leader and the group members explore the issue and attempt to find solutions.

Participants are not pressured to discuss their relative. Denial and resistance unfold gradually with the development of trust. Nonjudgmental support and education lead to understanding and open participation as family members learn some of the causes and cures of mental illness and substance disorders. This process parallels engagement and interventions developed for patient groups.

Emphasis is placed upon understanding discrete, multiple disorders. Some people believe that their relative drinks alcohol or uses drugs because he or she is mentally ill. This leads to seeking help for the mental illness alone with the expectation that the addiction will simply clear up. Others are uncertain that their relative has a mental illness and may perceive drinking and drug use as the cause of symptoms. Another common belief is that drinking or drug use as a leisure activity is the best quality of life a person with a severe mental illness can expect. Family members are taught the necessity of treatment, support, and relapse prevention for each disorder.

The supportive nature of the group process includes assisting each participant to consider his or her own well-being and separateness. As participants discuss their situations, leaders assist them to consider their personal well-being. Group members are encouraged to be supportive of one another, and to share their successes as well as their concerns.

Through this process, participants learn the parameters of their ability to be helpful to the dually diagnosed family member. This provides options for families to consider as they choose how they will expend their energy and resources.

Educational Content

Each meeting includes an informational component with use of videos, written materials, and guest speakers. Topics are addressed from many different perspectives and discussion from each member is encouraged. Some topics include: 1) The physiological aspects of the addictions, including effects upon brain chemistry; 2) Risk factors in mixing psychotropic medication with illicit substances; 3) Etiology of addictive disorders, including genetic and acquired factors; 4) Tolerance levels and other addictive syndromes; 5) The parallels between addictive disorders and mental illness; 6) Treatment methods and recovery from addictive disorders; 7) Special treatment programs for dually diagnosed persons; 8) Interaction effects of mental illness and addictive disorders; and 9) The impact of addictive disorders upon the family system.

It is most important for families to learn that the addictions are diseases that require treatment. Of particular importance is the understanding of the physical aspect of addictions. Without the knowledge that a relative may be responding to a physical addiction, families and providers frequently view substance abuse as a behavior that can be changed at will. This results in unrealistic expectations and frustrating, disappointing interactions.

ASSESSMENT OF FAMILIES

Assessment of families is an ongoing process. The following are some areas that need to be explored during initial contacts and continually updated throughout the entire process.

1. Assessment should include the **readiness** of the family to accept that their relative has an addictive disorder (and in some cases a mental illness), and the readiness of the patient to receive treatment. Interventions and content of the meetings will assist participants to reach the next step along the continuum of acceptance. Education about each disorder is directed toward dispelling stigma, shame, and guilt. Each of these areas parallel the process developed for patient groups. Discussions about the experiences families have in coping with or assisting their relative often validates the educational information and the disease concepts. When the dually diagnosed relative is discussed, his or her readiness to engage in treatment is determined.

2. Of extreme importance is the assessment of the **safety** of all concerned. Physical cravings for illicit substances can lead to various inappropriate behaviors in order to obtain money to buy drugs. Violence in families of substance abusers who are not diagnosed with a mental illness is well documented (Gorney, 1989; Gelles & Strauss, 1988). As is true with substance abuse, people tend to minimize, rationalize, and deny violence due to stigma, fear, and shame (Gorney, 1989). In a survey of NAMI members, 38 percent of the sample reported that their mentally ill relative was sometimes or frequently assaultive and destructive in the home (Swan & Lavitt, 1986). Families in our Maryland study reported violence (36%) and suicidal ideation (59%) as acute symptoms evoked by substance abuse.

In MICAA-NON groups, the unfolding of denial about assaultive and destructive behavior occurs in the same way that denial unfolds about other issues. In addition to the development of trust, participants learn from the media and from one another that these behaviors are common and symptomatic. This helps to alleviate shame and guilt. Families will then reveal the degree of discomfort they experience when their relative is under the influence of alcohol or drugs. Some members will describe past physical altercations or verbal threats. Leaders must consider whether or not there is an imminent danger. If there is, crisis intervention, hospitalization or alternative living arrangements may be recommended.

Lefley (1987-b) has written about "Aging Parents as Caregivers of Mentally Ill Adult Children." This may reflect the family compositions of some dually diagnosed people. With this family composition, the stressors may be manifold, and dangers more imminent.

3. Assessment of a **physical addiction** provides important information necessary to pursue an appropriate course of action. Questions about the dually diagnosed relative's drug(s) of choice, frequency and quantity of use, and length of time used (Sciacca, 1990) will facilitate this assessment. Families with physically addicted relatives come to understand the limitations of willful change and the treatment necessary for detoxification and recovery. Education about withdrawal effects and neurochemical and nutritional depletion are examples of information that helps families to understand the physical addictions.

4. It is important to explore the family's **support network**. This should include the quality of relationships between all family members; the identification of particular family members who provide

support and caregiving; and the presence or absence of outside supports including the relationships between the family and providers to the dually diagnosed patient. Assisting family members to increase supports for the family and the dually diagnosed relative is a formative goal. Leaders may attempt to engage other family members to attend MICAA-NON. Participants of MICAA-NON are encouraged to join their local AMI chapter. MICAA-NON meetings usually include members of AMI who will assist in engaging new AMI members.

Al-Anon speakers are invited to speak at MICAA-NON meetings. They are asked to discuss their relationships with addicted relatives and to answer questions about Al-Anon. Attending Al-Anon meetings can provide additional support for participants who have learned the similarities and differences between dually diagnosed persons and those with addictive disorders alone.

Participants are encouraged to communicate with those who provide treatment to their dually diagnosed relative. This includes asking questions and discussing their concerns.

5. It is important to assess the **family history of addictive disorders**. An assessment developed for dually diagnosed patients (Sciacca, 1990) details the family history of substance abuse and the patient's history. This provides information necessary to determine the possibility of genetic factors involved in the addictive disorders as well as acquired factors. The family dynamic of guarding information about family substance abuse, and experiences of betrayal when revealing it, exists for dually diagnosed patients and their families. As participants learn the symptoms of addictive disorders they may begin to question whether or not there is substance abuse among other family members.

Educating families about genetic research in alcoholism (Goodwin, 1985), which utilizes the same paradigms and yields results comparable to genetic research in schizophrenia (Torrey, 1983), is often easily understandable. As discussed in Chapter 5, other parallels between mental illness and substance disorders include treatments necessary to bring active symptoms into remission, the potential for relapse, and the need for ongoing support for continued remission for each disorder (Sciacca, 1991). Assisting families to recognize the addictions as a family disease, when relevant, can provide the clarity necessary to end years of misplaced blame and uncertainty.

Attention to the issues of dual diagnosis comes and goes as a priority in various states and communities. Advocacy sometimes consists of an individual family member who persistently tries to educate and influence entire bureaus, agencies, and other families (Sciacca, 1993). Successful efforts have resulted in educational presentations, and in some cases, education and training for providers in their communities. Efforts to develop services must include assisting families and patients to move from frustration and uncertainty to a stance of informed advocacy. This transition needs to take place for program administrators and providers of all services as well. Advocates for patients who are dually diagnosed must join together to form a cohesive group and a sustained effort to achieve the success that NAMI has achieved in helping those who have a mental illness alone.

REFERENCES

Al-Anon Family Groups. (1987). Al-Anon Family Group Headquarters, Inc., New York.

Evans, K., & Sullivan, J.M. (1990). *Dual Diagnosis: Counseling the Mentally Ill Substance Abuser*. New York: Guilford.

Gelles, R.J., & Strauss, M.A. (1988). *Intimate Violence*. New York: Springer.

Goodwin, D.W. (1985). Alcoholism and Genetics, The Sins of Fathers. *Archives of General Psychiatry. 42*, 171–174.

Gorney, B. (1989). Domestic Violence and Chemical Dependency: Dual Problems, Dual Interventions. *Journal of Psychoactive Drugs. 21*(2), 229–238.

Grosser, R.C., & Vine, P. (1991). Families as Advocates for the Mentally Ill: A Survey of Characteristics and Service Needs. *American Journal of Orthopsychiatry. 61*(2), 282–290.

Hatfield, A.B. (1990). *Family Education in Mental Illness*. New York: Guilford.

Hatfield, A.B. (1992). *Dual Diagnosis: Substance Abuse and Mental Illness*. Arlington, VA, National Alliance for the Mentally Ill.

Kashner, T.M., Rader, L., Rodell, D., Beck, M., Rodell, D., Beck, C., & Miller, K. (1991). Family Characteristics, Substance Abuse and Hospitalization Patterns of Patients With Schizophrenia. *Hospital and Community Psychiatry. 42*, 195–197.

Lefley, H.P. (1987-a). The Family's Response to Mental Illness in a Relative, In A.B. Hatfield (Ed.). *Families of the Mentally Ill: Meeting the Challenges, New Directions for Mental Health Services. 34*, San Francisco: Jossey-Bass.

Lefley, H.P. (1987-b). Aging Parents as Caregivers of Mentally Ill Adult Children: An Emerging Social Problem. *Hospital and Community Psychiatry. 38*, 1063–1070.

Marsh, D.T. (1992). *Families and Mental Illness: New Directions in Professional Practice.* New York: Praeger.

Minkoff, K., & Drake, R. (1991). "Editor's Notes," Dual Diagnosis of Major Mental Illness and Substance Disorder, ed. K. Minkoff and R. Drake. *New Directions for Mental Health Services.* San Fancisco: Jossey-Bass, No. 50, Summer, pp. 1–2.

Ridgely, M.S., Goldman, H.H., Willenbring (1990). Barriers to the Care of Persons with Dual Diagnosis: Organizational and Financing Issues. *Schizophrenia Bulletin, 16*(1), 123–132.

Sciacca, K. (1987-a). New Initiatives in the Treatment of the Chronic Patient with Alcohol/Substance Abuse Problems. *TIE Lines, 4*(3), pp. 5–6.

Sciacca, K. (1987-b). Alcohol/Substance Abuse Programs in New York State Psychiataric Centers Develop and Expand. This month in: *Mental Health (New York State Office of Mental Health). 10*(2)6.

Sciacca, K. (1989). MICAA-NON, Working with Families, Friends, and Advocates of Mentally Ill Chemical Abusers and Addicted (MICAA). *TIE Lines. 6*(3), 6–7.

Sciacca, K. (1990). *MIDAA Service Manual: A Step by Step Guide to Integrated Treatment, Program Development and Services for Multiple Disorders.* Sciacca Comprehensive Service Development for MIDAA, New York.

Sciacca, K. (1991). An Integrated Treatment Approach for Severely Mentally Ill Individuals with Substance Disorders. In K. Minkoff & R.E. Drake (Eds.), Dual Diagnosis of Major Mental Illness and Substance Disorder. *New Directions for Mental Health Services, 50*, pp. 69–84, San Francisco: Jossey-Bass.

Sciacca, K. (1993). Tennessee Encourages New Program Models for Multiple Disorders, Mental Illness, Drug Addiction and Alcoholism (MIDAA). *Curriculum and Training Network News,* Arlington, VA: NAMI, Vol. 3, Iss. 1, Spring 1993.

Steinwachs, D., Kasper J., & Skinner E.A. (1992). Family Perspectives on Meeting the Needs for Care of Severely Mentally Ill Relatives: A National Survey, Johns Hopkins University, Baltimore MD, 1992 (mimeo).

Swan, R.W., & Lavitt, M.R. (1986). Patterns of Adjustment to Violence in Families of the Mentally Ill. New Orleans, Elizabeth Wisner Research Center, Tulane University School of Social Work. 1986.

Torrey, E.F. (1983). *Surviving Schizophrenia, A Family Manual.* New York: Harper & Row.

U.S. News and World Report. When Mental Illness Hits Home. April, 24, 1989, pp. 55–65.

13

Housing for Persons with Chronic Mental Illness and Substance Use Disorders

LISA DIXON and FRED OSHER

INTRODUCTION

Access to appropriate housing is a critical component of care for persons with co-occurring mental illnesses and substance use disorders. Providers of treatment to these individuals must consider the frequent residential instability and homelessness of the dually diagnosed population. Studies focusing on persons with dual diagnoses have shown that, as a group, they are disproportionately at risk for housing instability and homelessness (Drake, Osher & Wallach, 1991-a). Epidemiologic studies have revealed that roughly 10% to 20% of homeless persons suffer from severe mental illnesses and co-occurring addictions (Tessler & Dennis, 1989; Drake, Osher & Wallach, 1991-a).

An aftercare study of patients of an urban state hospital revealed that over one-fourth of all patients studied and over one-half of patients with dual diagnoses had unstable housing and were at least temporarily homeless during the six months post-discharge (Drake et al., 1989-a). Another study of discharged state hospital patients found that 36% of patients experienced homelessness within six months of their discharge (Belcher, 1989). Patients who used alcohol and/or other drugs were more likely to experience homelessness. Drake, Wallach, Teague, Freeman, Paskus and Clark (1991-b) found that this phenomenon is not restricted to urban locations. They studied housing instability of patients with schizophrenia in a rural area where patients had extensive family supports and low-cost housing was available. This study found that co-occurring disorders were strongly correlated with housing instability and that the majority of patients with schizophrenia and alcohol problems experienced housing instability during a six-month period.

Thus, alcohol and/or drug use by persons with severe mental illness must be considered as a high risk behavior for homelessness. This is critical because homelessness and housing instability can exacerbate addiction and mental illness, creating a malignant cycle of increased symptomatology, disability and exposure to harsh living environments.

WHY ARE PERSONS WITH DUAL DIAGNOSES AT RISK FOR HOMELESSNESS?

Although the association of housing instability with dual diagnoses has not been comprehensively researched, a number of systemic, legal and clinical issues may contribute to this finding.

Systemic Issues

Systemic barriers to *clinical care* for persons with dual diagnoses have been well-documented. Lack of a common administrative structure for alcohol, drug and mental health services at the Federal, State, and local levels, scarce resources, historic distrust and philosophical conflicts between providers of addiction services and mental health services, as well as separate funding streams for treatment of both disorders have contributed to the problem (Ridgely, Goldman & Willenbring, 1990). The nature of these problems and potential solutions are discussed elsewhere in this volume.

As a result of administrative divisions, many residential treatment programs for persons with mental illness specifically bar patients with co-occurring substance abuse problems. Residential addiction programs similarly bar patients with a co-occurring mental illness. The locus of responsibility for providing housing and clinical services to homeless persons with dual diagnoses is also unclear and variable at different localities; the question is raised of whether mental health providers, substance abuse providers or providers of housing services should be responsible for assuring access to housing?

Legal Issues

Legal issues present obstacles to housing for persons with dual diagnoses. The Fair Housing Amendment of 1988 extended protections of Federal fair housing legislation to people with disabilities, including persons with mental illness. Practically speaking, persons with dual diagnoses face discriminatory treatment. Individuals with histories of drug dependence are not eligible for public housing programs unless they are receiving addiction treatment (Mental Health Law Project, 1989). As mentioned above, addiction treatment for the individual with dual diagnoses may be unavailable or inappropriate. Thus, persons with dual diagnoses may be shut out of the very housing programs for which they are eligible due to disabilities associated with drug and/or alcohol use. In addition, many potential landlords might reject persons involved with illicit drugs due to liability issues (Drake et al. 1991-a).

Homeless persons with dual diagnoses have been shown to have greater histories of arrest when compared to homeless persons without dual diagnoses. The lack of an adequate treatment system for persons with dual diagnoses may lead to arrest rather than to an appropriate referral to a treatment facility. These arrests are frequently for misdemeanors due to bizarre symptoms and erratic behavior, publicly displayed because of their lack of shelter, rather than more severe criminal acts (Abram & Teplin, 1991). Once having an arrest record, it may be more difficult for persons with dual diagnoses to obtain housing of any kind.

Clinical Issues

Persons with dual diagnoses have been found to have greater rates of psychotic symptoms (Negrete, Knapp, Douglas & Smith, 1986), non-compliance with treatment (Osher et al., submitted), psychiatric hospitalizations (Safer, 1987), and violent, disruptive behavior (Safer, 1987; Abram & Teplin, 1991) including suicide (Drake, Osher & Wallach, 1989-b; Caton, 1981; Dassori, Mezzich & Keshavan, 1990) than persons with mental illnesses only. It is not surprising, then, that individuals with this clinical profile would have trouble accessing housing and be at risk for losing housing. Families, already under stress from coping with mental illness, may be unable to tolerate the additional disruption, and perhaps danger, associated with co-occurring substance abuse, resulting in eviction from the family home (Robinson, Dixon, Stewart, Harold & Lehman, 1993). Other residential settings, such as board and care homes or public housing settings, may also be unable to tolerate the erratic behaviors of persons with dual diagnoses, their disturbance of other tenants, or their unreliable rental payments. Frequent or prolonged hospitalizations may result in loss of housing placement, particularly in locations where affordable housing is scarce and waiting lists are common.

An additional important consideration is that persons with dual diagnoses may be unable to manage income or benefits, particularly if such funds are used to support a drug or alcohol habit. Consequently, there is no money for rent and other bills; the street, hospital, or prison become the only other shelter alternatives. The use of a representative payee can partially remedy this problem, but many persons with dual diagnoses are not engaged enough with a provider who can assess the need for a representative payee and follow through with the laborious paperwork involved. Even if the need for a representative payee is obvious, it can be extremely difficult to find persons willing to serve as payees for these individuals.

Finally, persons with dual diagnoses may be unable to succeed at therapeutic drug treatment communities designed for persons with substance dependence alone. The interpersonal intensity and confrontation often built into such programs may be intolerable to individuals with dual diagnoses. Overall, the clearest predictor of success in traditional alcohol and drug treatment setting is the patient's degree of psychiatric severity; more severe psychiatric illness has been associated with less successful outcomes following alcohol and drug treatment (McClellan, Luborsky, Woody, O'Brien & Druley, 1983).

CLINICAL STRATEGIES

Given the vulnerability of individuals with dual diagnoses to homelessness, the next question is how to modify clinical strategies to treat
homeless or marginally housed persons with these co-occurring disorders. Clinicians must have an adequate understanding of the basic
principles of treating persons with dual diagnoses. As discussed elsewhere in this volume, an integrated treatment program organized
around treatment phases — engagement, persuasion, active treatment and relapse prevention (Osher & Kofoed, 1989) — has gained
widespread acceptance. Successful programs have recognized the
need to attend to both disorders, persisting through multiple crises
and relapses, utilizing educational and supportive groups, and in
many cases providing comprehensive case management services.

It is also essential to know about the specific characteristics of
homeless persons with dual diagnoses in order to develop treatment
strategies. In a review of ten federally funded epidemiologic studies
of homelessness, Fisher (1990) found that individuals with dual diagnoses were more likely to be older and male and less likely to be
employed compared with homeless persons without dual diagnoses.
Individuals with dual diagnoses as well as persons with alcoholism
had longer durations of homelessness and were more likely to be
local residents than were other subgroups of homeless persons.
Dually diagnosed people experienced harsher living conditions,
such as living on the streets rather than in shelters (Fischer &
Breakey, 1990), had greater health difficulties, and received more
services than other subgroups (Fisher, 1990). Increased levels of
psychological distress and demoralization, greater likelihood of
granting sexual favors in exchange for food and money, and increased police contact and incarceration have been associated with
homeless persons who have mental illness and alcoholism compared
with other homeless groups (Koegel & Burnam, 1987). Dually diagnosed people were also less likely to have contacts and receive help
from their families, and like homeless persons with alcoholism, were
highly prone to victimization. Isolation, mistrust of people and institutions, and resistance to accepting help were characteristic of
homeless persons with dual diagnoses (Blankertz, Cnaan, White, Fox
& Messinger, 1990; Drake et al., 1991-a).

The available evidence thus reveals the severity and intensity of
the problems experienced by dually diagnosed homeless people.
Modifications of treatment and housing strategies used for domi-

ciled persons with dual diagnoses will be discussed in terms of the phases of treatment mentioned above and special considerations for homeless persons.

Engagement: Homelessness complicates the already difficult engagement phase in the treatment of individuals with severe mental illness and substance use disorders. Assertive and prolonged outreach is essential, as clients in this phase generally do not come to the program office or keep appointments. Lack of money for transportation, the daily demands of obtaining food and shelter, psychiatric symptoms, ongoing substance use and associated organic deficits may cause clients to miss appointments. Since clients often have limited access to phones and mail, tracking clients requires tenacity and familiarity with the streets, knowledge of where homeless people tend to congregate, as well as extensive contacts with homeless providers in the community.

Providing for basic needs such as clothes, showers, and food may be helpful in the engagement process. The promise of safe, clean housing may motivate clients to enter the treatment system. Provision of badly needed material resources can help to draw clients into a trusting relationship where staff can persuade them to enter treatment for substance abuse and/or mental illness and help them identify other long term goals.

The engagement process for homeless persons with dual diagnoses is likely to include the need for crisis intervention. These crises, whether they be psychiatric, medical, or related to housing, may provide important opportunities to engage the client by addressing their acute needs. Crises, while facilitating the engagement process, may require that difficult clinical decisions be made with very little information about the client beyond the immediate need.

Ms. G, a homeless dually diagnosed woman, had refused to engage with a treatment system for many years before presenting at a day shelter in a moderately agitated state. An outreach team was called. The physician immediately recognized that the woman was jaundiced, an indication of liver disease associated with alcoholism. The patient's psychosis interfered with her obtaining necessary medical and psychiatric treatment. The physician filed an emergency petition. The patient was experiencing a medical and psychiatric crisis, and the physician had to make a rapid assessment without full knowledge of the patient's situation and the potential clinical impact of the petition.

The decision had to made quickly because the patient was about to leave the shelter.

While hospitals and detoxification centers may serve as initial points of entry into treatment, often crises have to be handled in the community, either because the situation is not acute enough to require hospitalization, clients refuse hospitalization, or local hospitals reluctantly admit homeless, indigent people. A treatment team needs to be able to access diverse housing or shelter options on an acute basis, since housing instability persists even after housing is obtained.

Staff and client security is another critical issue, especially during the engagement phase when little may be known about the client. Streets and shelters are often dangerous, and use of drugs and alcohol is associated with crime and victimization. Clients may feel that carrying a weapon is necessary for self-protection. Clinicians and programs must set limits and ensure safety without compromising their ability to provide services. At one extreme, programs might have metal detectors at the office entrance. While providing more assurance that clients will not bring weapons into the office, such a practice might inhibit clients from accessing services. At the other extreme would be a total disregard for the potential that clients may be carrying weapons. Each program must consider its situation and needs, make appropriate policies, and train staff well in how to prevent dangerous situations.

Assessment of homeless individuals with dual diagnoses can be especially difficult. Assessment must be ongoing and well integrated into the engagement phase. Potential clients do not come to programs carrying an updated medical chart. Referrals often come from shelter staff along with general comments about the client's needs. A client's psychiatric symptoms and cognitive deficits may hinder the ability of the provider to obtain accurate historical information. Usually homeless people are not self-referred and may be suspicious of treatment providers and unwilling to provide much personal information. The identification of family, friends, and previous providers, information critical to the assessment process, may not occur in the early stages of engagement. Information about histories of violence, suicide attempts, and medical problems are especially important to obtain. Lack of this information may result in the necessity for staff to develop interim treatment plans without knowing the optimal clinical approach and potential dangers.

Another aspect of assessment which must not be ignored is the possibility of HIV infection. Homeless persons with dual diagnoses are at increased risk for HIV infection. The use of disinhibiting substances, cognitive impairment, and the high prevalence of HIV seropositivity among homeless persons are significant risk factors for the spread of HIV infection. In addition, homelessness might lead to increased difficulty obtaining clean needles, prostitution involving multiple partners, or rape. Where there is no accessible medical clinic, programs may need to provide their own HIV testing and counseling, as a part of a comprehensive attempt to meet medical and social needs.

Persuasion: Persuasion involves reducing a patient's denial about a mental illness and/or substance abuse problem. Success can be measured by a patient's acknowledgement that a problem exists and by the commitment to pursue active treatment. In addition to the persuasion strategies for dually diagnosed clients mentioned elsewhere in this volume, the linkage of housing opportunities to abstinence should be emphasized in persuading homeless dually diagnosed people to enter active treatment. Providers should review with clients how substance use has influenced their housing opportunities in the past and point out how access to current housing options is limited by ongoing drug use.

The use of representative payeeship assumes special importance in working with homeless persons with dual diagnoses in the persuasion phase. Implicit in the condition of homelessness is that the client's basic needs are not being met. Although there may be a multitude of reasons for this, (e.g., the absence of decent affordable housing,) the only way to stop the cycle of homelessness and drug use may be for the program, family or some other individual to assume the responsibility of managing the person's finances.

A responsible representative payee cannot only assist individuals in meeting basic needs, but also can provide some interpersonal stability in the consistent relationship with the payee. If this responsibility is handled sensitively and with respect, giving the client as much independence and control as possible, the persuasion process can be facilitated. If patients relapse and require hospitalization and detoxification, or simply spend some time on the streets, there is at least a home to which they can return if the rent is paid. Such a service may need to be offered as part of an overall treatment and support intervention. The establishment of a representative payee fits best in the persuasion phase; it may alienate individuals during the engagement phase and may be absolutely necessary for active treatment to proceed.

An issue related to using representative payees is employment of other strategies which patients may experience as coercive in nature. The frequent legal entanglements of homeless dually diagnosed persons offer opportunities for clinicians to utilize the requirement for court-ordered treatment. The clinician's attitude and approach in this context can be critical. There is clearly an obligation to honor court-ordered requirements. There may also be significant clinical utility in pursuing these obligations. Concrete requirements with direct consequences for failure to meet these conditions may be an important way to persuade people to begin treatment. This coercive approach is *not* a substitute for treatment and will likely be ineffective if successful treatment does not ensue. Nevertheless, legal requirements may be an effective way to stop the cycle of homelessness, mental illness and addiction. Future research may reveal the extent to which structure and rules are themselves therapeutic at different phases of treatment of persons with dual diagnoses.

Mr. J, a 43 year old black man, had a diagnosis of schizophrenia, alcoholism, and mild mental retardation. He had multiple psychiatric hospitalizations and a history of numerous arrests for offenses almost uniformly associated with his drinking. He acknowledged that his longest period of sobriety had been just a few months. After an arrest for assault, he was found not criminally responsible and court-ordered for psychiatric treatment. While Mr. J was required to stay in an inpatient setting, the treatment team repetitively pointed out that his drinking led to the arrest which led to his hospitalization. He was able to connect these events. A simple, concrete treatment program was then set up requiring that Mr. J take Antabuse supervised by mental health staff during the week and shelter staff on weekends. It was made very clear to Mr. J that if he missed even one dose of Antabuse or any of his appointments, he would have to return for inpatient treatment. Mr. J succeeded with over a year of sobriety. He was able to articulate the need to stop drinking. The court-ordered requirement for treatment faciliated the persuasion and then active treatment of Mr. J.

Active Treatment: In the active treatment phase, patients develop the skills and relationships necessary to achieve and maintain sobriety and minimize disabilities associated with their mental illness. The basic strategies useful in this phase are discussed elsewhere in this volume and include individual and group therapy, education and rehabilitation. Mental health programs serving homeless persons with dual diagnoses in particular may need to develop addiction treatment services internally. External referrals may fail because of the inability of the client to develop trust with another treatment system or program. Imposing such a transition without very close follow-up might result in the client falling out of care. Further, it is often difficult to refer homeless clients to traditional mental health and substance abuse programs, either because the programs will not admit them or because the services may be inappropriate to their needs. Programs serving homeless people must either be prepared to provide active treatment within their own program or to extend continued support to the client as they begin active treatment in another agency.

It is especially important to recognize that the older homeless dually diagnosed person may have more organic deficits, possibly associated with long-term use of alcohol or drugs. This might require that cognitive and educational approaches to treatment receive less emphasis than behavioral approaches with support. Patients with alcohol-induced dementia in addition to a schizophrenic or mood disorder may not understand or be able to articulate the idea that drinking causes multiple problems in their lives, but might develop sobriety with material, emotional and behavioral support.

Mr. W, a 58 year old white man, had been homeless for many years. He had a long history of heavy alcohol use, multiple episodes of head trauma, as well as a diagnosis of schizophrenia. Upon referral for treatment, tuberculosis was diagnosed. Mr. W was hospitalized for six months while receiving anti-tuberculosis therapy. While hospitalized, he did not have access to alcohol, was stabilized on antipsychotic medication, and was found eligible for SSI payments. Psychological testing revealed a significant dementia. Upon discharge, Mr. W rented a room, had supervision and assistance with money managment from treatment providers, and maintained his sobriety. He occasionally would acknowledge that he knew it was better to drink "sodas" than to drink alcohol, but this knowledge seemed less important to maintaining his sobriety than the structure and emotional support he was receiving.

Relapse Prevention: Both addiction and mental illness tend to be relapsing disorders. Addiction specialists refer to the concept of on-going "recovery" rather than cure. The relapse prevention phase focuses on minimizing the extent of and damage due to patient relapse. The lack of social and family supports of the homeless individual with dual diagnoses may lead to increased fragility and greater vulnerability to relapse, both in terms of addiction and mental illness. Relapse may then lead to another episode of homelessness — the cycle begins anew. It is thus especially important for programs and clinicians to plan for this phase and offer continued treatment and support.

HOUSING STRATEGIES

Housing strategies for homeless or marginally housed persons with dual diagnoses must be developed in tandem with clinical strategies. Development of housing strategies requires consideration of types of housing, associated support, organization and funding. In addition to the factors important for housing of any citizen such as preference, safety, and convenience, special attention must be paid to the substance use and mental illness of the person with dual diagnoses.

Newman (1992) describes two different philosophies which have been organizing principles for housing programs for severely and persistently mentally ill persons. The first, more traditional program, utilizes a "level of care" or "continuum" approach. The varying needs of the heterogeneous mentally ill population are addressed by offering several settings, each with different levels of service and supervision as well as restrictiveness (Ridgeway & Zipple, 1990). A second model has been called the "supported housing" model. In this model, the intensity of supported services varies with client need while the residential site remains the same.

The expectation of the level of care model is that clients "advance" to more independent, less supervised and less restrictive settings as they master the appropriate skills required at their current placement. Lengths of stay may be limited at each placement. Examples of different levels provided in one community might include a quarterway house, a halfway house, supervised apartments, and independent living (Ridgeway & Zipple, 1990).

This model has been criticized for a number of important reasons (Newman, 1992). The requirement that individuals change housing as they "progress" through the continuum may be counterproductive, even causing symptomatic relapse. Further, since there are no data on how rapidly a given individual should progress through the phases, time limits seem arbitrary and a step-wise progression may not mirror the client's clinical course. Specific residences designated for persons with mental illness may also make their integration into the community more difficult, and they may encounter stigma, discrimination and community opposition. Consumers have also complained about the institutional qualities of many treatment-oriented housing settings and the fact that consumer choice or preference may be ignored (Harp, 1990).

The supported housing model views housing primarily as a place to live, not to receive treatment. Central to this model is the coupling of consumer-chosen housing with the flexible provision of whatever individual services and assistance that individual may need to maintain that housing choice. Proponents of this model emphasize that it facilitates normal community roles, social integration, and increased independence and control for the client (Ridgeway & Zipple, 1990). Studies of this model and its cost are underway (Newman, 1992).

While some view these models as mutually exclusive, the authors and others believe that supported housing is important part of the continuum of residential housing of which the goal is to help patients to move from the hospital into the community (Fields, 1990). For persons with dual diagnoses, housing choice may be limited by community alternatives. This selection should be made in part by an assessment of the clinical needs of the individual. It may vary depending on what phase of treatment the person is in and what support needs exist.

A critical question for persons with dual diagnoses is whether treatment can or should be separated from housing. This question presents a practical clinical problem. So-called wet housing, or housing in which the use of drugs and alcohol is tolerated, may be the only housing choice acceptable to the patient in the early phases of engagement and treatment. Yet, some clinicians believe that allowing substance use in housing sustains, or "enables" use and is countertherapeutic. At the same time, the achievement and maintenance of sobriety may be unlikely, if not impossible, without adequate housing (Drake et al. 1991-a). Some patients may be motivated to stop using drugs if they are aware that their housing depends on their sobriety. Other patients will continue to use despite prohibitions, will get evicted, and wind up on the streets in circumstances which are not conducive to pursuing sobriety. The solution to this dilemma is vexing and will require experimentation with different models and client choices.

At the present time, most housing options sponsored by mental health or substance abuse providers are "dry housing," or housing where alcohol and drug use is prohibited. Perhaps a continuum of care should provide for "degrees of dryness." Some have even proposed the concept of *damp housing*, where there is an expectation of abstinence on the premises, but clients are not required to agree to be abstinent off-site. At one end of the housing continuum could be shelters and other "safe havens" that are very tolerant of use while towards the other end of the continuum could be stronger expectations and limits.

What levels of structure, supervision and support with housing are effective for persons with dual diagnoses? In a discussion of the Robert Wood Johnson Foundation-HUD Demonstration Program on Chronic Mental Illness, Newman (1992) noted, "It is particularly difficult to serve active substance abusers and those with recent histories of destructive behaviors using an independent housing strategy." The engagement phase might require flexible housing regulations while intensive and assertive supportive services are provided. High levels of structure and supervision may be unacceptable to persons during engagement. However, once engagement is achieved, clients might tolerate a greater degree of structure and supervision during the persuasion and active treatment phases when peer interaction and clear limits may be therapeutic. Less structure and supervision consistent with supported housing models may be more appropriate during later phases of treatment such as the relapse prevention phase. Preliminary data from a project conducted in Washington, D.C. suggests that homeless dually diagnosed persons did not succeed in a supported housing model until they were in the active treatment phase (Drake, personal communication). However, access to permanent housing with ongoing support will be the goal for most clients.

SPECIAL CONSIDERATIONS FOR HOUSING DUALLY DIAGNOSED INDIVIDUALS

Shelterization

The phenomenon of "shelterization" refers to a process of acculturation and adaptation that homeless people who utilize shelters may experience (Gounis & Susser, 1990, Grunberg & Eagle, 1990). This process, while helping homeless persons cope with their surroundings in the short-run, may impede the process of moving out of the shelter system which becomes a social community with familiar social rules. Some formerly homeless clients may experience loneliness when they transition from the noisy, busy shelter system to independent housing. There is some evidence that more intensive support during the transition from shelter to housing may result in increased residential stability (Center for Mental Health Services, 1994). If programs attend to these needs, as well as clinical needs, housing stability will be enhanced.

Tolerance and Safety

As mentioned above, homeless individuals are frequently victims of crime, and life on the streets is wrought with danger. Consideration of this fact is essential in planning housing for persons with mental illness who have drug addiction problems. Housing must be safe, whether a transitional shelter with a time-limited stay, a group home with other residents with mental illness, or an independent apartment fully integrated into the community. On the other hand, providers must be tolerant of the adjustment process required of homeless persons as they leave the dangers of the streets and shelters. It may take some time and experience for these individuals to feel safe.

Client Preference

In making choices about housing, programs must balance housing availability, client preferences and client needs. Most people prefer independent housing. They do not always succeed at this choice (Center for Mental Health Services, 1994). Clients with active addiction problems may prefer independent living, but have previous experience suggesting they need more structure and supervision. Dixon, Krauss, Myers and Lehman (1994) have shown that it was possible to honor the housing preferences of the majority of homeless mentally ill patients treated in their program which had a limited number of Section 8 certificates. Programs should try to accommodate client choices and provide the extra supports that may be necessary to make the various housing options work.

Cooperative Agreements Between Providers and Housers

Given the complex and varied requirements of providing housing and clinical care as well as the historic administrative and economic separation of these two services, it makes sense for mental health/substance abuse providers and housing providers to agree prospectively to work together. Otherwise, there is considerable danger that patients will fall between the cracks, receiving housing without mental health and addiction services or visa versa. Cooperative agreements should outline the respective roles and responsibilities of housing providers, mental health providers and substance abuse providers. The specific details of such an agreement will need to reflect community resources. The common goal will be to maintain individuals with dual diagnoses in the community.

The following case illustrates some of the points we have mentioned above including the difficulty of engagement, the importance of attending to patient choice, and the need to take a comprehensive approach to patients' needs.

Mr. R is a 40 year old black man referred to a program designed for homeless persons with mental illness while he was in the psychiatric hospital. He had a diagnosis of schizophrenia and a history of drug abuse including intravenous drugs. He had never been in any sustained treatment in the past and had been living on the streets for at least 10 years at the time of referral.

Mr. R met the treatment team and was intially superficially cooperative and agreeable to working with the team. The next day, he eloped from the hospital while at an activity. HIV testing obtained in the hospital revealed that the patient was HIV positive. A member of the team who was familiar with the shelter system tracked the patient down a few days later. The patient was impressed at the persistence of the team. He expressed no interest in housing, but was pleased to come to the office each day to shower and wash his clothes. He was initially uninterested in medication because of a history of severe side effects, but expressed the desire to avoid the hospital. The team convinced him that medication would help him in this goal. He took a low dose of antipsychotic medication each day when he came in for his shower. Mr R did not feel that he had a current alcohol or drug problem, but acknowledged using such drugs from time to time. He was already aware of his HIV status, but refused to obtain any medical treatment. Initially, Mr. R did not wish to obtain any income through benefits. However, over the ensuing few months, Mr. R agreed to apply for public assistance for which the team was the patient's payee.

By the end of the first year, the team had won the patient's trust. He had not been rehospitalized and had kept himself clean and neat. During the second year of treatment, the patient applied and was approved for social security income due to his psychiatric disability. The team was the patient's payee for this income given the patient's ongoing substance use. He began to attend substance use treatment groups within the program, and to speak spontaneously about the need to stop using drugs and alcohol. He also agreed to use part of his income to pay for a room and to attend the HIV clinic for somatic services.

While Mr. R still uses drugs and alcohol, his use has apparently been reduced enough through working with the treatment team that he is no longer homeless, avoids the hospital, and receives the medical services he needs. His quality of life has improved, and he reports being more satisfied with his circumstances.

CONCLUSION

While models for providing housing to individuals with co-occurring disorders have not been fully explicated and evaluated, reducing the morbidity and mortality associated with homelessness for these persons is critical. Dually diagnosed people who are homeless or at risk for homelessness have special needs and characteristics that must be considered when planning treatment. Common principles must guide approaches to this population until empirical data are available. These include: individualized housing and treatment planning must be derived from thorough assessments; flexibility and creativity must outweigh intolerance and categorical programs; and the development of ongoing therapeutic relationships must be established over time.

REFERENCES

Abram, K.M., & Teplin, L.A. (1991). Co-occurring disorders among mentally ill jail detainees. *American Psychologist. 46*, 1036–1045.

Belcher, J.R. (1989). On becoming homeless. A study of chronically mentally ill persons. *Journal of Community Psychology. 17*, 173–185.

Blankertz, L., Cnaan, M.R., White, K., Fox, J., & Messinger, K. (1990). Outreach efforts with dually diagnosed homeless persons. Families in Society. *The Journal of Contemporary Human Services. 71*, 387–395.

Caton, C. (1981). The new chronic patient and the system of community care. *Hospital and Community Psychiatry. 32*, 475–478.

Center for Mental Health Services (1994). *Making a Difference: Interim Status Report of the McKinney Demonstration Program for Homeless Adults with Serious Mental Illness.* Rockville, MD: Substance Abuse and Mental Health Services Administration.

Dassori, A.M., Mezzich, J.E., & Keshavan, M. (1990). Suicidal indicators in schizophrenia. *Acta Psychiatrica Scandinavia. 81*, 409–413.

Dixon, L., Krauss, N., Myers P., & Lehman, A.L. (1994). Clinical and treatment correlates of access to Section 8 certificates for homeless mentally ill persons. *Hospital and Community Psychiatry. 45*, 1196–1200.

Drake, R.E., Osher, F.C., & Wallach, M.A. (1991-a). Homelessness and dual diagnosis. *American Psychologist. 46*, 1149–1158.

Drake, R.E., Wallach, M.A., Teague, G.H., Freeman, D.H., Paskus, T.S., & Clark, T.A. (1991-b). Housing instability and homelessness among rural schizophrenic patients. *American Journal of Psychiatry. 148*, 330–336.

Drake, R.E., Wallach, M.A., & Hoffman, J.S. (1989-a). Housing instability and homelessness among aftercare patients of an urban state hospital. *Hospital and Community Psychiatry. 40*, 46–51.

Drake, R.E., Osher, F.C., & Wallach, M.A. (1989-b): Alcohol use and abuse in schizophrenia: A prospective community study. *Journal of Nervous and Mental Disease. 177*, 408–414.

Fields, S. (1990). The relationship between residential treatment and supported housing in a community system of services. *Psychosocial Rehabilitation Journal. 13*, 105–113.

Fischer, P.J. (1990). *Alcohol and drug abuse and mental health problems among homeless persons: A review of the literature.* 1980–1990. Rockville, MD: National Institute on Alcohol Abuse and Alcoholism and National Institute of Mental Health.

Fischer, P.J., & Breakey, W.J. (1990). The epidemiology of alcoholism in a homeless population: Findings from the Baltimore homeless study. Paper presented at the 16th Annual Alcohol Epidemiology Symposium of the Kettil Bruun Society for Social and Epidemiological Research on Alcohol, Budapest, Hungary.

Gounis, K., & Susser, E. (1990). Shelterization and its implications for mental health services. In Cohen, N. (Ed). *Psychiatry Takes To the Streets: Outreach and Crisis Intervention for the Mentally Ill*. New York, The Guilford Press.

Grunberg, J., & Eagle, P.F. (1990). Shelterization: How the homeless adapt to shelter living. *Hospital and Community Psychiatry. 41*, 521–525.

Harp, Howie. (1990). Independent living with support services: The goal of future for mental health consumers. *Psychosocial Rehabilitation Journal. 13*(4), 85–89.

Koegal, P., & Burnam, M.A. (1987). *The epidemiology of alcohol abuse and dependence among the homeless: Findings from the inner city of Los Angeles.* Rockville, MD: National Institute on Alcohol Abuse and Alcoholism.

McClellan, A.T., Luborsky, L., Woody, G.E., O'Brien, C.P., & Druley, K.A. (1983). Predicting response to alcohol and drug abuse treatments: Role of psychiatric severity. *Archives of General Psychiatry. 40*, 620–625.

Mental Health Law Project. (1989). *The impact of the fair housing amendments on land-use regulations affecting people with disabilities*. Washington, DC.

Negrete, J.C., Knapp, W.P., Douglas, D.E., Smith, W.B. (1986). Cannabis affects the severity of schizophrenic symptoms: Results of a clinical survey. *Psychological Medicine. 16*, 515–520.

Newman, S.E. (1992). *The Severely mentally ill homeless: Housing Needs and Housing Policy*. The Johns Hopkins University Institute for Policy Studies, Occasional Paper No. 12, Shriver Hall, Baltimore Maryland.

Osher, F., Drake, R., Noordsy, D., Teague, G.E., Hurlbut, S.C., Biefanz, S.C., & Beaudett, M.S. (1994). Correlates and outcomes of alcohol use disorder among rural outpatients with schizophrenia. *Journal of Clinical Psychiatry. 3*, 109–113.

Osher, F.C., & Kofoed, L.I. (1989). Treatment of patients with psychiatric and psychoactive substance abuse disorders. *Hospital and Community Psychiatry. 40*, 1025–1030.

Ridgely, M.S., Goldman, H.H., & Willenbring, M. (1990). Barriers to the care of persons with dual diagnoses: Organizational and financing issues. *Schizophrenia Bulletin. 16*, 123–132.

Ridgeway, P., & Zipple, A.M. (1990). The paradigm shift in residential services: From the linear continuum to supported housing approaches. *Psychosocial Rehabilitation Journal. 13*, 11–31.

Robinson, C.T., Dixon, L., Stewart, B., Harold, J., Lehman, A.F., (1993). Family connections of the homeless mentally ill, Poster Session, 146th Annual Meeting of the American Psychiatric Association, San Francisco, CA.

Safer, D. (1987). Substance abuse by young adult chronic patients. *Hospital and Community Psychiatry. 38*, 511–514.

Tessler, R.C., & Dennis, D.L. (1989). A synthesis of NIMH-funded research concerning persons who are homeless and mentally ill. Rockville, MD: National Institute of Mental Health, Division of Education and Service System Liaison.

14

"Double Jeopardy": Legal Issues Affecting Persons with Dual Diagnoses

LAURA M. CHAMPLAIN and STANLEY S. HERR

INTRODUCTION

Individuals with dual diagnoses[1] frequently face a type of "double jeopardy" in their contacts with the legal system. Many of these individuals require support and advocacy to meet their everyday needs and to protect their legal rights. The combined stigma of mental illness and substance abuse, however, can lead to bias and discrimination, barring access to necessary and appropriate services and resulting in inadequate and substandard representation. This "double jeopardy" frequently arises when an individual's rights and liberty are abridged, as in a criminal or civil commitment context. However, with access to advocacy and information about their rights, these individuals can overcome injustice as well as obtain affirmative benefits and legal protection.

With the aid of legal and other professionals, dually diagnosed individuals have secured rights under Social Security, housing, family, non-discrimination, and other laws. The Americans with Disabilities Act of 1990 (ADA)[2] and the Rehabilitation Act of 1973 (Rehabilitation Act)[3] can open new avenues to opportunity. For example, qualified individuals with mental and physical disabilities now enjoy the same rights to employment, public accommodations, and public services as other Americans. Nevertheless, a person's addiction to, or abuse of, illegal drugs and/or alcohol may affect that person's eligibility for benefits, services, access to public accommodations, or employment under these laws. Service providers — whether in doctor's offices or other health facilities — must also comply with the ADA to uphold their patients' rights and to avoid legal liability.

Some homeless persons with dual diagnoses come into contact with the legal system because of criminal activity. The combination of mental illness, substance abuse, and a transient lifestyle can cause behavioral problems that often lead to illegal activity and petty non-violent crimes. In theory, when the dually diagnosed offender with serious impairments enters the criminal justice system, a competency determination must be rendered by the court. Often, this evaluation can take weeks while the homeless defendant waits in jail. Throughout the evaluation process, lack of appropriate treatment can further complicate the alleged offender's mental and drug or alcohol abuse problems. In practice, lawyers often bypass this potentially destructive process by not raising incompetency claims for clients of questionable capacity.

The array of legal issues affecting persons with dual diagnoses is as diverse as the population itself. No chapter can encompass all the issues they share with persons who need mental health care,[4] social security disability benefits,[5] or fair tenant-landlord relations.[6] For example, the Clinical Law Office of the University of Maryland School of Law has represented such persons in unemployment benefits hearings, federal disability determinations, managed healthcare hearings, guardianships, civil commitment proceedings, and class-action suits to secure the right to effective treatment in community-based settings. This chapter is intended to provide an introduction to some novel as well as recurrent issues facing people at risk of this type of double jeopardy. Advocacy — formal and informal, systemic and individual-focused — will be required to resolve those issues.

ASSERTING THE DUALLY DIAGNOSED INDIVIDUAL'S AFFIRMATIVE RIGHTS

Selected Provisions of the Rehabilitation Act of 1973 and the Americans with Disabilities Act

Congress enacted the ADA in 1990 in order to guarantee the civil rights of individuals with disabilities. The legislation adopted many of the key antidiscrimination provisions and concepts of the Rehabilitation Act of 1973, and fully extended prohibitions of disability-based discrimination to the private sector. The 1973 law protects individuals with disabilities from discrimination by the federal government,[7] private employers contracting with the federal government,[8] and federally assisted programs.[9] Under Section 504 of the Rehabilitation Act, for example, a handicapped[10] individual cannot be excluded from participation in any program or activity that receives Federal financial assistance or be subjected to discrimination solely on the basis of a handicap.[11] By providing the foundation for implementing regulations enacted by all federal agencies, the Rehabilitation Act is a basic civil rights act for persons with disabilities.[12] Employers, public universities, and other federally aided programs are required to make a reasonable accommodation for an individual's disabilities unless it would cause an undue hardship to the operations of the business or program.[13] The Rehabilitation Act does not set absolute rules, but rather requires an individualized approach that determines the existence of discrimination on a case-by-case basis.[14]

Like the Rehabilitation Act, the ADA also addresses discrimination in employment, public services and transportation, public accommodations, and telecommunications.[15] The ADA proposes to "provide clear, strong, consistent, and enforceable standards"[16] that will enable individuals with disabilities to integrate fully into American society.[17]

Title I, which deals with employment discrimination, is one of the most far-reaching of the ADA provisions and could have the greatest impact on dually diagnosed individuals. Unlike the Rehabilitation Act, the ADA covers the private sector. It initially applied to all businesses with 25 or more employees,[18] and then extended to smaller businesses with 15 or more employees as of July 26, 1994.

Although the ADA declares that an employer may not "discriminate against a qualified individual with a disability because of that disability,"[19] Title I excludes certain categories of drug users and alcoholics from receiving protection. Under the ADA, a disability is broadly defined as "(a) physical or mental impairment that substantially limits one or more of the major life activities of such individual; (b) a record of such impairment; or (c) being regarded as having such an impairment."[20] Mental impairments can include some learning disabilities, mental retardation, and psychiatric illness. To constitute a disability, any impairment must substantially limit a major life activity such as learning, self-care, walking, breathing, hearing, or working.[21] The impairment must be serious, not a typical limitation or the result of a temporary illness or accident that people commonly experience.[22]

The second part of the definition applies to individuals with a record of such an impairment. This section protects individuals who have a history of, or have recovered from a mental illness or who were misdiagnosed as mentally retarded.[23] The ADA also applies to individuals who are treated as disabled by their employers even though they are not limited in their ability to perform other major life activities.[24] A person with controlled high-blood pressure who is assigned to a less strenuous job, is an example of a person within this definition of disability. So is a person with a facial scar or burn who is screened-off from customers because of a feared or perceived negative reaction.[25]

Even if an individual has a disability that meets the defined criteria, the individual must be "qualified" in order to be covered under the ADA. A "qualified individual with a disability" means a person who can perform the essential functions of that person's current job or the job being sought, with or without reasonable accommodation by the employer.[26] In some cases, dually diagnosed individuals may face problems in establishing themselves as a "qualified individual with a disability." For example, any applicant or employee who is a current user of illegal drugs is not covered under the ADA if the employer makes an employment decision on the basis of the drug use.[27]

The ADA provides the employer with several options to combat illegal drug use and alcohol abuse. Before discussing these options, it will be helpful to look at the status of persons who use drugs and alcohol under Section 504 of the Rehabilitation Act and the accompanying case law.

The Status of Persons Who Abuse Substances under the Rehabilitation Act

Neither the Rehabilitation Act of 1973 nor its legislative history specifically addressed whether substance abusers were protected from discrimination. To clarify this point, the U.S. Department of Health, Education and Welfare (later redesignated the Department of Health and Human Services) requested that the U.S. Attorney General issue an advisory opinion.[28] In 1977, Attorney General Griffen Bell decided that alcoholism and drug addiction were intended to be covered within the definition of handicapped individuals because both were generally considered to be diseases that impaired major life activities.[29] He advised, however, that this conclusion did not "necessarily entitle [substance abusers] to full coverage [under] section 504 [since it] protected only 'qualified' handicapped individuals."[30]

Under this new ruling some employers feared that they would be obligated to hire substance abusers in order to meet the requirement of the statute.[31] In response to inquiries from employers and in an effort to clarify the Attorney General's opinion, Congress passed the Rehabilitation, Comprehensive Services, and Developmental Disabilities Amendments of 1978 (1978 Amendments).[32] The 1978 Amendments narrowed the definition of "handicapped individual" to exclude alcoholics and/or drug abusers whose current substance abuse prevents them from "performing the duties of the job" or whose drug or alcohol use "would constitute a direct threat to property or the safety of others."[33] The substance abuser was now protected as a handicapped individual, but only if he or she was qualified to perform the job in question.[34]

Case Law Applying The Rehabilitation Act

Precedent clearly establishes that substance abuse is a "handicap" for purposes of the Rehabilitation Act.[35] The cases that protect substance abusers involve former or recovering alcoholics and drug addicts.[36] In *Burka v. New York City Transit Authority*,[37] the U.S. District Court extensively analyzed the legislative history behind Section 504 and the 1978

Amendments, concluding that "section 504 protects only those otherwise qualified drug abusers who have been or are being rehabilitated. It does not protect the illegal narcotics abuser who has not sought or is not seeking treatment for his or her condition."[38] The court determined that the Congressional intent behind the 1978 Amendments was not to broaden the coverage of Section 504 "beyond rehabilitated and rehabilitating drug abusers."[39]

The Supreme Court upheld a Veterans Administration (VA) regulation in *Traynor v. Turnage*[40] that would deny benefits to veterans whose alcoholism was not the result of a psychiatric disorder. In 1977, the Congress extended the ten-year period in which veterans could use their educational benefits if the delay was caused by a "physical or mental disability which was not the result of willful misconduct."[41] Under the VA regulations, primary alcoholism (alcoholism that is not the result of a psychiatric disorder) constituted willful misconduct.

The Supreme Court perceived no conflict between the VA regulation and Section 504. Rather, the Court held that nothing in the Rehabilitation Act "requires that any benefit extended to one category of handicapped persons also be extended to all other categories of handicapped persons."[42] Veterans who are denied the opportunity to extend their eligibility for benefits are not denied "'solely by reason of their handicap' but because they engaged with some degree of willfulness in the conduct that caused them to become disabled."[43] The Court refused to rule on whether alcoholism is a disease that cannot be voluntarily controlled and concluded that this was an issue better left to Congress.[44] Instead the Court simply decided that the two regulations were not incompatible and that there could be some distinction between behavior that causes alcoholism and the condition of being an alcoholic.[45]

Teahan v. Metro-North Commuter Railroad Co.[46] presents an intriguing case study of the willingness of the judiciary to protect substance abusers once they seek treatment. During most of his five years of employment with Metro-North (1983–1988), John Teahan actively abused alcohol and drugs, a condition that led to numerous unexcused absences from work. On December 28, 1987, Teahan voluntarily entered a substance-abuse rehabilitation program. He did so just prior to receiving a letter from his employer charging him with excessive absenteeism. Teahan successfully completed the 30-day rehabilitation program and returned to work on January 28, 1988.

Metro-North continued to pursue Teahan's dismissal and fired him on April 11, 1988 even though he had no absences and fully performed his job after completing the program.[47]

Teahan sued the railroad alleging that his dismissal violated Section 504 of the Rehabilitation Act because as a drug and alcohol user he was an "otherwise qualified individual with handicaps" who had been fired "solely by reason of" his handicap. Although the U.S. District Court upheld the dismissal, the U.S. Court of Appeals reversed since Metro-North had relied on Teahan's absenteeism as the basis for his dismissal and these absences were shown to be causally related to his handicap as a substance abuser.[48]

In this case, the court reasoned that employers cannot be allowed to discriminate by basing dismissal on the manifestation or symptom of a disability. When the employer relies on the disability or its manifestation to terminate an employee, *Teahan* holds that the "'solely by reason of' element is by definition satisfied. The question then becomes whether the employee is qualified despite his or her handicap to perform the essential functions of the job."[49] If the employee is not qualified for the position, then the dismissal is not discriminatory. However, an employer cannot justify termination based on conduct caused by the handicap (for example, the thumping noise that an employee with a limp might make) without giving the employee the chance to demonstrate his or her qualifications for the job. In Teahan's case the court held that if the dismissal is based on absenteeism and the absences are caused by the substance abuse, the employee is terminated "solely by reason of" the handicap and is entitled to demonstrate that he is "otherwise qualified" for the position.

This case also generously decides in favor of substance abusers in determining who is a "current" substance abuser. The legislative history behind the Rehabilitation Act supports the court's decision that the relevant time for an assessment of Teahan's status was the time of his actual firing (April 1988 when he had apparently recovered), not the earlier date when the decision to seek termination was made. The statute was specifically written to ensure that rehabilitated or rehabilitating substance abusers are protected from discrimination based on past substance abuse. Thus, an employee's substance abuse problem must be "severe and recent enough so that the employer is justified in believing that the employee is unable to perform the essential duties of the job" in order for the employer to exclude the individual from Section 504 coverage.[50] These are obviously fact-sensitive issues, requiring remand to the trial court to gauge the likelihood of relapse, to determine if Teahan was otherwise qualified for his job, and to judge whether his dismissal was justified.

Provisions of the ADA Pertaining to Drug and Alcohol Use

When Congress passed the ADA, the Bush administration had adopted a policy of so-called "zero-tolerance" for illegal drug use. In the spirit of that policy, the ADA modified the protection granted under the Rehabilitation Act to substance abusers.[51] It removed an employee or applicant from the definition of a "qualified individual with a disability" if that individual is "currently engaging in the illegal use of drugs, when the covered entity acts on the basis of such use."[52] It also barred from the Rehabilitation Act's protection an "individual who is an alcoholic whose current use of alcohol prevents such individual from performing the duties of the job in question."[53]

If an employer takes action based on an individual's substance abuse and not because of some other physical or mental impairment, the individual with alcohol or drug abuse is not covered under the ADA. This provision is particularly important for dually diagnosed individuals because they are only entitled to the protection of the ADA if their employer discriminates on the basis of their mental disability. Therefore, a current drug or alcohol addiction constitutes an impediment to obtaining the law's antidiscrimination protection. The ADA, however, does include a provision that covers rehabilitated or recovering substance abusers. It defines a qualified individual with a disability as including someone who:

> (1) has successfully completed a supervised drug rehabilitation program and is no longer engaging in the illegal use of drugs, or has otherwise been rehabilitated successfully and is no longer engaging in such use; (2) is participating in a supervised rehabilitation program and is no longer engaging in such use; or (3) is erroneously regarded as engaging in such use, but is not engaging in such use.[54]

As our discussion of the *Teahan* case noted, Congress adopted this definition to protect individuals who are attending a rehabilitation program so that they need not fear losing their jobs and to encourage other substance abusers to seek treatment.[55] The judiciary has interpreted this statute as plainly designed to "protect rehabilitated or rehabilitating substance abusers from retroactive punishment by employers" and to forestall discharge based on "past substance abuse problems that an employee has presently overcome."[56]

The ADA also provides protection to employers by granting them considerable latitude when dealing with individuals who use illegal drugs. Specifically, the ADA permits employers the following: to prohibit all employees from using illegal drugs or alcohol at the workplace, to require that employees not be under the influence of illegal drugs or alcohol at the workplace, to require that employees conform to the Drug Free Workplace Act, and to meet the same standards of job performance and behavior that other employees are required to meet.[57] Furthermore, if an employee is fired or an applicant is denied a job because of a positive drug test for an illegal substance, that individual has no protection under the ADA.[58]

Case Law Applying the ADA and the Fair Housing Amendments Act

Because parts of the ADA only became effective in 1992, the courts have decided few cases relying solely on its provisions. These early decisions have emphasized the need for individualized assessment of the litigant's disabilities and the importance of avoiding blanket types of disqualification due to rigidity or stereotyping. Cases decided under the Fair Housing Amendments Act of 1988 (FHAA)[59] may provide an indication of how persons with dual diagnoses will fare in litigation brought under the ADA.[60] In 1992, the U.S. Court of Appeals for the Fourth Circuit held in *U.S. v. Southern Management Corporation*[61] that a current user of illegal drugs was not to be considered a handicapped person under the FHAA because the definition of a handicapped individual was "not intended to be used to condone or protect illegal activity."[62] Since the FHAA defines handicap in terms identical to the Rehabilitation Act, it is not surprising that the court opined that "individuals who have a record of drug use or addiction but who do not currently use illegal drugs would continue to be protected if they fell under the definition of handicap."[63]

Summary of Protection Under the ADA

Whether under the FHAA or the ADA, current use of illegal drugs bars any statutory protection. The status of alcoholics is more favorable since illegal consumption is not involved. They are disqualified from statutory coverage if shown to be unable to perform the duties of their jobs, but not merely on the basis of status. The ADA seeks to strike a balance between the needs of employers to maintain a drug and alcohol-free workplace and the rights and interests of employees with substance abuse related or other disabilities.[64]

Consequently, advocates and service providers have yet another reason to help their addicted clients become involved in treatment or rehabilitation. Even though these individuals may have a defined mental impairment, the law's "zero-tolerance" provisions could provide employers with a basis to deny employment. An alcoholic person with a mental disability would be in a similar position if use of alcohol degraded the performance of essential job functions or made the individual a threat to the safety or property of others.

Dually diagnosed people who begin rehabilitation or who have successfully completed a treatment program are covered under the ADA and should assert their rights to be fairly evaluated in employment situations. An employer cannot discriminate against a dually diagnosed applicant or employee if that person is qualified for the position. Moreover, the employer is required to make a reasonable accommodation to adjust to the individual's disability as long as it does not create an undue hardship to the employer's business. Advocates can defend these rights both formally (through administrative complaint or litigation) or informally (through negotiation and counselling) with both the dually diagnosed individual and the potential or current employer. To remain covered by the rights established by the ADA, however, dually diagnosed clients must conform their behavior to reasonable workplace norms to satisfy the legal standard of a "qualified individual with a disability."

CRIMINAL JUSTICE AND INDIVIDUAL RIGHTS OF DUALLY DIAGNOSED CLIENTS

As discussed in Chapter 13, many dually diagnosed individuals face the additional problem of homelessness or a transient lifestyle. This unstable environment can lead to contact with the criminal justice system, both as an offender and as a victim. Frequently criminal offenses fall into the category of petty nonviolent minor crimes — such as shoplifting, vagrancy, trespassing, disorderly conduct, prostitution, public drunkenness, and disturbing the peace.[65] A combination of mental illness and substance abuse can produce behavioral problems that result in deviant and often illegal activity.[66] In addition, several cities and towns have enacted rules and laws that prohibit the homeless from begging, loitering, or sleeping in parks or on the streets.[67] As a result, the homeless can face arrest or harassment for simply trying to survive on the streets — an already hostile environment.

Empirical studies demonstrate that homeless persons tend to be charged with nonviolent offenses. However, they also tend to be charged with more severe offenses than domiciled persons or to be arrested for incidents that would not result in the arrest of those with homes.[68] As one student of this topic notes, there may even be a tendency on the part of police investigators to focus on homeless shelters, recalling "the gendarme's command in *Casablanca*, to 'round up the usual suspects.'"[69] Among homeless men, a Texas study showed that only 1% of their arrests were for violent crimes against people and 20% of their arrests charged serious crimes against property such as burglary, arson, or car theft. The vast majority of incidents (78%) were for minor infractions such as liquor or drug violations or disorderly conduct.[70]

Once arrested, the dually diagnosed person confronts a series of problems. Many jurisdictions find it easier or less expensive to incarcerate mentally ill persons who abuse substances than to find appropriate treatment facilities or obtain hospitalization.[71] If the court or counsel questions an alleged offender's competency, a special hearing may be ordered to decide if the person can stand trial. Although this initial evaluation may be held promptly, if the state cannot establish that the accused is competent or requires treatment to become competent, further competency tests are required.[72] The court has the option to try to place the individual in a hospital pending the results of the additional tests, but an inadequate supply of hospital beds often means that the dually diagnosed person will wait in jail.[73] This wait can last several weeks and can mean that the mentally ill defendant or substance abuser spends more time in jail than if formally charged with a minor crime.[74] While in jail, the dually diagnosed person frequently does not receive needed treatment, which often complicates existing mental health problems.[75] Defense lawyers for such individuals charged with minor crimes may strategically avoid raising a competency issue, preferring to minimize risks of their client's loss of liberty.

If such cases come to trial, a host of difficult legal issues may be encountered. *Does the individual have the requisite intent to commit a crime?* Courts have split as to whether a homeless individual discovered in a vacant building or other unauthorized space can be charged with burglary rather than the less serious charge of trespass.[76] *Is homelessness a proper factor in mitigation?* One court spared a "homeless wanderer who had been in and out of mental institutions for the past four to five years" from the death penalty, reasoning that a competent but homeless mentally ill person did not deserve to die and sentenced him to life without the possibility of parole.[77] Some judges seem to have sentenced homeless defendants more harshly than others.[78] Many of these defendants have not been well-served by revolving-door mental commitments, or closed doors when they sought treatment on their own. In one particularly poignant example, a homeless man, "wandering, cold and scared, about the city seeking shelter" broke into a building after he was denied admission at a county mental health facility.[79]

Vigorous and systemic multi-disciplinary advocacy is needed to confront these chronic institutional failures. For instance, advocates for dually diagnosed defendants should seek speedier evaluation processes to enable their clients to receive the appropriate treatment and care for their mental illness and substance abuse problems.[80] On a broader scale, clinicians, social workers, other mental health professionals, and legal advocates can work for greater communication and cooperation between the criminal and mental health systems in order to direct dually diagnosed offenders to proper treatment.[81] Likewise, they can educate communities and legislatures about the need for additional mental health facilities and drug and alcohol treatment programs to help dually diagnosed individuals become functioning members of society.[82] Most important, advocates can seek to ensure that the individual rights of mentally ill substance abusers are protected and that society treat their behavior rather than criminalize it.

ADVOCATING FOR DUALLY DIAGNOSED CLIENTS

Effective advocacy can make a critical difference in the lives of dually diagnosed individuals by assisting them in obtaining access to services, by protecting their legal rights, and by empowering them to make decisions and to exercise greater control over their lives.[83] Dually diagnosed and mentally disabled clients, however, routinely fall prey to a "double jeopardy" whereby some of the neediest clients receive substandard representation or no representation as a result of their inability to obtain access to advocates.[84] This hazard can occur when an attorney substitutes his/her goals or objectives for the client's, treats the disabled client with paternalism and insensitivity, or when attorneys lack the skill or desire to counsel and communicate effectively with their client.

Over the past several decades, confusion and controversy have governed the representation of individuals with disabilities. The legal profession's Model Code of Professional Responsibility offers little guidance to practitioners for such clients.[85] The newer Model Rules of Professional Conduct[86] do state that attorneys shall maintain as normal a client-lawyer relationship as reasonably possible with mentally impaired clients.[87] However, an attorney may use discretion to evaluate the nature of the relationship with the client and may "seek the appointment of a guardian or take other protective action with respect to a client, only when the lawyer reasonably believes that the client cannot adequately act in the client's own interest."[88] Consequently, in a client-centered approach to lawyering, the attorneys would maintain their loyalty to the client's interest and objectives while seeking to empower the client through communication and joint decision-making as much as reasonably possible.

This type of approach can sometimes bring lawyers and clinicians into conflict, particularly when they disagree about the objectives and goals of the client/patient and how to meet those objectives. Each group should remain cognizant that they are both working to achieve what is in the best interest of the dually diagnosed individual. The stigma of mental illness and substance abuse can leave these clients open to discrimination in qualifying for housing, public benefits, treatment, and employment. By working together, clinicians and advocates can assist these clients in overcoming the "double jeopardy" that they too often encounter.

Test cases and other forms of impact litigation pose opportunities for such collaboration. For example, the recent appellate opinion in *Heard v. Cuomo*[89] heralds the potential sweeping effects that successful advocacy can produce for a group of homeless, mentally ill persons. John Heard and a class of similarly situated homeless persons sued the state of New York and the New York City Health and Hospitals Corporation (HHC) for not fulfilling their duties under the

Mental Hygiene Law. Those duties specifically required the provider system to implement individual written service plans for mentally ill patients and find them adequate and appropriate housing upon discharge from the hospital.[90] The evidence at trial showed that plaintiff Heard was repeatedly released from city hospitals with nothing more than two subway tokens and referral to a shelter.[91]

On February 18, 1993, New York's highest court affirmed a lower court decision that could potentially force New York City to provide additional housing for homeless mentally ill people. The Court of Appeals ruling requires HHC to "take concrete steps to prescribe in the [written] discharge plan the specific type of adequate and appropriate housing necessary for the about-to-be discharged mentally ill patients; to assist in locating such adequate and appropriate housing before [discharge] ...; to discharge the patients in accordance with their individual written service plans that include the recommended housing; and to coordinate the effectuation of those efforts among the responsible entities."[92] Justice Bellacosa, writing for the unanimous court, declared that while neither the statute nor the court's judgement required HHC to build, create, or pay for housing, the statute demanded more than aspirations of cooperation and altruism. In insisting on incremental action, the court reasoned that "HHC is obligated to give some real legal and practical teeth to this task so that ... the statutory mandate is not rendered illusory."[93]

Heard's case is a classic instance of a judicial declaration of rights that properly leaves the details of implementation and finance to the relevant political and professional actors. The trial court acknowledged that determining the means to carry out the statutory requirements is "left to the agencies involved."[94] Legal advocates for homeless people with disabilities accomplished the initial task of securing the litigants' rights under the Mental Hygiene Law and putting "the force of law behind the promise of community mental health."[95] Now, a combined effort by the public, politicians, attorneys, social workers, and clinicians must take up the fight to ensure that resources are made available and used effectively to secure housing and services. Only then will the rights of vulnerable persons receive authentic protection.

Inspired advocacy will continue to be essential to preserving individual and collective rights. This need is magnified by unbalanced journalism,[96] adverse public opinion, and mounting threats of legislative or executive rollbacks.[97] In August 1994, for example, Congress exacted a limit of 36 months on the payment of Social Security disability benefits based on alcoholism or drug abuse.[98] Bitterly opposing this cutoff, the advocates succeeded in wresting such concessions as 1) having medical benefit continue after the 36-month period as long as the disability and its need for treatment exist and 2) for Social Security Disability Insurance (SSDI) recipients, having the limitation period start from the month after the individual begins rehabilitation treatment.[99] Advocates also face challenges at the state level, such as Maryland's proposed abolition of the Disability Assistance and Loan Program (DALP), which provides a subsidence cash payment, medical assistance, and advocacy help to quality for SSI benefits. Although individuals with dual diagnoses comprise only a minority of DALP recipients, their needs will likewise be affected by the sudden cutoff of benefits, whose predicted consequences include increased homelessness and health care costs.[100]

Legal advocates, social workers, and other clinicians may need additional guidance and support from a variety of national, state, and local organizations to resolve such critical legal problems of the dually diagnosed patient. Every state has a federally funded agency established for the protection and advocacy of recipients of mental health services.[101] Likewise, the legal services offices of the National Legal Services Corporation, state bar association committees on the needs of persons with disabilities, the American Bar Association Commission on Mental and Physical Disability Law, and the clinical law programs of local law schools are all good reference sources. Washington-based public interest law firms, such as the Bazelon Center for Mental Health Law, are also resources for law reform and technical assistance. Clinicians must reach out to lawyers to help their patients in legal and social distress.

CONCLUSION

Dually diagnosed persons face particular hardships in obtaining needed services because they bear the double stigma of mental illness and substance abuse. Often, this stigma can lead to denials of affirmative rights, access to services, and representation for some of the neediest individuals in society. This kind of "double jeopardy" can be diminished with effective advocacy and support by legal and clinical professionals. New legal tools are available for this purpose. Specifically, the Americans with Disabilities Act, along with other state and federal legislation, can open doors that have been closed to many persons with disabilities.

Both informal and formal advocacy can aid dually diagnosed people in securing their rights under these laws. Advocates can guide such individuals through the maze of administrative agencies, assist them in securing benefits, and connect them to appropriate treatment facilities and service providers. Lawyers can use litigation and formal advocacy, if necessary, to protect a client's rights, whether it be in a commitment hearing, an administrative procedure, a civil court, or a criminal proceeding. Clinicians must also engage in lobbying and legislative advocacy to safeguard such individuals' rights and interests in an era of budgetary cuts by federal, state, and local governments. They must ensure access to effective treatment as a crucial factor in the patient's survival and rehabilitation. Advocates of all types must alert government officials to the complex issues affecting individuals with dual diagnosis and the need to preserve funding for treatment programs and benefits that assist persons with dual disabilities. Likewise, coalitions of consumers, clinicians, and advocates must be vigilant to save and expand these resources. In the current climate of conservatism, such disability-action coalitions are more vital than ever.

The results of this active support and advocacy will be measured by the successful integration of dually diagnosed individuals in society; it will be measured by each patient who gains access to treatment programs, housing, public services, and employment. Sensitive, caring, and effective representation can ensure that an individual's substance abuse and mental illness do not bar him or her from enjoying the same rights as other Americans.

NOTES

1. The term *individuals with dual diagnosis* refers to individuals diagnosed with two separate disorders. For purposes of this chapter, people with both mental illness and a substance abuse problem are considered dually diagnosed individuals.
2. Pub. L. No. 101-336, 104 Stat. 327 (codified in 29 U.S.C. §706 and 42 U.S.C. §12101 et seq. (1990)) [hereinafter ADA].

3. Pub. L. No. 93-112, 87 Stat. 357 (codified in 29 U.S.C. §§701–724, 730–732, 740, 741, 750, 770–776, 780–787, 790–794 (1973)) [hereinafter Rehabilitation Act].

4. For a manual for clinicians, see S. Herr, S. Arons, and R. Wallace, *Legal Rights and Mental Health Care*. Lexington, Mass.: Lexington Books (1983).

5. See D. Sweeney and J. Lyko, *Practice Manual for Social Security Claims*, New York: Practicing Law Institute (1980); H. McCormick, *Social Security Claims and Procedures*, vol. 1 (3d ed. 1983).

6. See Mental Health Law Project, *Rights of Tenants with Disabilities Under the Fair Housing Amendments Act of 1988*. Washington, DC: Author (1989).

7. 29 U.S.C. §791.

8. *Id*. §793.

9. *Id*. §794.

10. The Rehabilitation Act uses the term handicapped to refer to individuals with disabilities. This terminology will appear throughout the text when referencing this act. Congress later chose to adopt the term disability instead of handicap because it reflects the current terminology preferred by most persons with disabilities.

11. 29 U.S.C. §794.

12. J. Parry, R. Reynolds, and D. Zuckerman, *Mental Disability Law: A Primer*. Washington, DC: American Bar Association Commission on the Mentally Disabled (3d ed. 1984).

13. In *Southeastern Community College v. Davis*, 442 U.S. 397 (1979), the Supreme Court decided that an accommodation is not reasonable if it imposes either "undue financial and administrative burdens" or requires "a fundamental alteration in the nature of the program." *Id*. at 410, 412.

14. The Supreme Court endorsed this approach in *School Board of Nassau County, Fla. v. Arline*, 480 U.S. 273 (1987).

15. 42 U.S.C. §§12111–12117, 12131–12134, 12141–12150, 12161–12165, 12181–12189 (1990).

16. *Id*. §12101 (b)(2).

17. Special Project, *Addiction as Disability: The Protection of Alcoholics and Drug Addicts under the Americans with Disabilities Act of 1990*, 44 Vand. L. Rev. 713, 714 (1991).

18. 42 U.S.C. §12111 (5)(A).

19. *Id*. §12112 (a).

20. *Id*. §12102 (2).

21. 28 C.F.R. § 36.104[2]; H.R. Rep. No. 485, 101st Cong., 2nd Sess. at 51–52.

22. The legislative history to the ADA offers the example of an individual who walks ten miles and then begins to experience pain on the eleventh mile. Because such pain would be typical for most people, the individual would not be considered to have an impairment. See H.R. Rep. No. 485, 101st Cong., 2nd Sess. at 51–52.

23. *Id.* at 52–53.

24. *Id.* at 53. See also *School Board of Nassau County, Fla. v. Arline*, 480 U.S. 273, 279 (1987) (teacher with tuberculosis protected under section 504 of the Rehabilitation Act because some impairments "might not diminish a person's physical or mental capabilities, but could ... limit that person's ability to work as a result of the negative reactions of others.").

25. Special Project, *supra* note 17, at 720. For a recent case decided on parallel state law disability discrimination grounds, see *Hodgson v. Mt. Mansfield Co.*, 624 A.2d 1122, 1129–32 (Vt. Sup. Ct. 1992) (maid whose lack of teeth is perceived by ski resort employer to be a visible physical impairment rendering her unfit for job involving customer contact is regarded by employer as a disabled individual).

26. 42 U.S.C. §12111 (8).

27. *Id.* §12114 (a).

28. Special Project, *supra* note 17, at 727.

29. 43 Op. Att'y Gen. No. 12 (1977).

30. Fitzpatrick, *Alcoholism as a Handicap Under Federal and State Employment Discrimination*, Advanced Employment Law and Litigation, American Law Institute (1991).

31. Special Project, *supra* note 17, at 728.

32. Pub. L. No. 95-602, 92 Stat. 2955 (1978)(codified in 29 U.S.C. §706 (1988)) [hereinafter 1978 Amendments].

33. *Id.*

34. Special Project, *supra* note 17, at 729.

35. *Id.*

36. *Teahan v. Metro-North Commuter Railroad Co.*, 951 F.2d 511, 517 (2nd Cir. 1991); *Whitlock v. Donovan*, 598 F. Supp. 126 (D.D.C. 1984)(rehabilitated alcoholics are covered by Section 504 of the Rehabilitation Act); *Wallace v. Veterans Administration*, 683 F. Supp. 758 (D. Kan. 1988)(recovering drug-addicted nurse was a handicapped individual and otherwise qualified within the meaning of the Rehabilitation Act of 1973); *Davis v. Bucher*, 451 F. Supp. 791 (E.D. Pa. 1978)(persons with a history of drug abuse, including individuals participating in methadone maintenance programs, fall within the protection of the Rehabilitation Act).

37. 680 F. Supp. 590 (S.D.N.Y. 1988).

38. *Id.* at 598.

39. *Id.*

40. 485 U.S. 535 (1988).

41. Pub. L. 95-202, Tit. II, §203(a)(1), 91 Stat. 1429, 38 U.S.C. §1662 (a)(1).

42. 485 U.S. 535, 549.

43. *Id.* at 550.

44. *Id.* at 552.

45. Fitzpatrick, *supra* note 30.

46. 951 F. 2d 511 (2nd Cir. 1991).

47. *Id.* at 513.

48. *Id.* at 517.

49. *Id.* at 516.

50. *Id.* at 519.

51. 42 U.S.C. §12114.

52. *Id.*

53. 29 U.S.C. §706(8)(C)(v).

54. 42 U.S.C. §12114 (b).

55. Special Project, *supra* note 17, at 736.

56. *Teahan*, 951 F.2d at 518.

57. 42 U.S.C. §12114 (c).

58. Fitzpatrick, *supra* note 30.

59. Pub. L. No. 100-430, 102 Stat. 1619 (codified in 28 U.S.C. §§2341–2342 and 42 U.S.C. §§3601–3602, 3604–3608, 3610–3619, 3631 (1988)) [hereinafter FHAA].

60. See, e.g., *Weintraub v. Board of Bar Examiners*, No. OE-0087 (Mass. Sup. Jud. Ct. July 2, 1992)(Massachusetts bar exam applicant with a learning disability granted double the time to take the bar exam as a reasonable accommodation that does not substantially alter the nature of the program); *Anderson v. Little League Baseball*, 794 F. Supp. 342 (D. Ariz. 1992)(coach in a wheelchair cannot be barred from serving as an on-field coach if League's safety concerns are based on "generalizations, stereotype, or unfounded fears"). For opinions under federal and state laws relating to employment discrimination based on disability, see Bureau of National Affairs. *Americans with Disabilities Cases*, vol. 1. Washington, DC: Author (1993).

61. 955 F.2d 914 (4th Cir. 1992).

62. *Id.* at 921.

63. *Id.*

64. Special Project, *supra* note 17, at 736.

65. U.S. Department of Health and Human Services, *Outcasts on Main Street, Federal Task Force on Homelessness and Severe Mental Illness*, at 11. Washington, DC: Author (1992).

66. *Id*. at 12.

67. See *Young v. New York City Transit Authority*, 903 F.2d 146 (2d Cir. 1990), *cert. denied*, 498 U.S. 984 (1990)(challenge to New York City Transit Authority rule that prohibited begging at all its facilities); *Papachristou v. City of Jacksonville*, 405 U.S. 156 (1972)(Supreme Court struck down a vagrancy statute because it encouraged an arbitrary and discriminatory enforcement of the law that impacted disproportionately on poor people); *Pottinger v. City of Miami*, 720 F. Supp. 955 (S.D. Fla. 1992)(homeless people cannot be arrested for conducting life activities, such as sleeping and cleaning themselves, in parks set aside as "sanctuaries").

68. Fischer, *Criminal Activity Among the Homeless: A Study of Arrests in Baltimore*, 39 Hospital & Community Psychiatry 46 (1988).

69. Kathryn Simpson, "Problems of the Homeless in the Criminal Justice System" at 5, Law and the Homeless Seminar paper, University of Maryland School of Law (Dec. 2, 1992).

70. *Id*. at 8 [citing Snow, Baker & Anderson, *Criminality and Homeless Men: An Empirical Assessment*, 36 Social Problems 532, 536–537 (1989), an Austin, Texas study comparing far higher arrest rates for domiciled men of 9.9% for violent crimes against persons, and 55.2% for serious crimes against property].

71. *Outcasts on Main Street, supra* note 65, at 11–12.

72. Pro Bono Coordinating Committee and University of Maryland School of Law, *Representing Homeless, Elderly, and Other Low-Income Persons: A Pro Bono Desk Manual*. Baltimore: MICPEL (1989) at §§11.9–11.10.

73. *Id*.

74. *Id*.

75. *Id*.

76. Compare *People v. Gaines*, 547 N.Y.S.2d 620, 622 (Ct. App. 1989) (no intent) with *State v. Chief Eagle*, 377 N.W.2d 141, 144, 147 (S.D. 1985) (intent to commit burglary for homeless man eating food in someone else's car, although dissenting opinion states that he "only wanted to get out of the cold").

77. *Haynes v. State*, 739 P.2d 497, 503 (Nev. 1987).

78. See, e.g., *People v. Williams*, 559 N.E.2d 96 (Ill. App. 1 Dist. 1990); *People v. Sehr*, 501 N.E.2d 848 (Ill. App. 2 Dist. 1986); and other cases collected in Simpson, *supra* note 69, 14–26.

79. E.g., *People v. Hoffman*, 208 Cal. Rptr. 609, 619 (Cal App. 4 Dist. 1984).

80. *Id*.

81. *Outcasts on Main Street, supra* note 65, at 11–12.

82. Siegel, *Homelessness: Its Origins, Civil Liberties Problems and Possible Solutions*, 36 Vill. L. Rev. 1063, 1082 (1991).

83. *A Pro Bono Desk Manual, supra* note 72, §7.

84. Herr, *Clients in Limbo: Asserting the Rights of Persons with Dual Disabilities, Mental Retardation and Mental Health: Classification, Diagnosis, Treatment, Services* 338–353 (J. Stark, F. Menolascino, M. Albarelli, V. Gray eds.). New York: Springer-Verlag (1988).

85. See American Bar Association, *Model Code of Professional Responsibility*, EC 7-11,7-12 Washington, DC: Bureau of National Affairs (1982).

86. American Bar Association, Model Rules of Professional Conduct, Washington, DC: Bureau of National Affairs (1983).

87. *Id.* Rule 1.14(a).

88. *Id.* Rule 1.14(b).

89. 80 N.Y.2d 684, 610 N.E.2d 348 (1993).

90. N.Y. Mental Hygiene Law §§ 29.15 (f)(g)(m)(n) (McKinney 1980).

91. Dugger, *Ruling Issued on Housing Mentally Ill*, N.Y. Times, February 19, 1993, at B1.

92. 80 N.Y.2d at 691.

93. *Id.* at 690.

94. *Id.* at 691.

95. Dugger, *supra* 91.

96. E.g., Haner and O'Donnell, *America's Most Wanted Welfare Plan: Addicts Squander Checks on Drugs and Alcohol*, Baltimore Sun, Jan. 23, 1995, 1A.

97. O'Donnell and Haner, *Drug Addicts, Alcoholics May Lose Federal Money*, Baltimore Sun, Feb. 9, 1995, 13A; Rich, *Congress Planning Cutoff for Addicts on Disability Rolls*, Washington Post, June 20, 1994, A1.

98. Social Security Independence and Program Improvements Act of 1994, Pub. L. No. 103-296, 108 Stat. 1464–1544 (1994).

99. In contrast, SSI recipients face a 36-month time period that begins from the date the individual becomes eligible for benefits. This law goes into effect with the disability checks mailed in March 1995.

100. Frece, *Advocates, Recipients Plead to Save Program: Glendening Targets Disability Benefits*, Baltimore Sun, Feb. 9, 1995, 1B.

101. Protection and Advocacy for Mentally Ill Act of 1986, 42 U.S.C. §10805 (1986).

15

Integrating Mental Health and Substance Abuse Treatments for Persons with Chronic Mental Disorders: A Model

ROBERT E. DRAKE, DOUGLAS L. NOORDSY,
and THEIMANN ACKERSON

INTRODUCTION

For historical reasons, the U.S. has two (and sometimes more) separate systems for mental health and substance abuse treatment. Programs within these two systems diverge in multiple aspects: different clinicians, education and training programs, credentialing systems, explantory models, treatment interventions, regulations, and reimbursement mechanisms. In contrast to this clear separation of treatment programs and providers, patients themselves have largely failed to acquire their disorders in pure culture — i.e., large proportions of those who receive treatment in either system have co-existing mental health and substance use disorders (Regier et al., 1990). Consequently, those with comorbid conditions are often treated in one system that does not adequately address the concurrent disorder or in parallel systems that are poorly coordinated.

As has been well documented by now, treatment of dual disorders in separate but parallel systems is inefficient and ineffective (Ridgely, Goldman & Willenbring, 1990). Treatment in parallel systems fails for a variety of reasons. Programs and clinicians in parallel systems do not modify their previous ways of working to accomodate comorbid conditions. Treatment in either system is incomplete due to inattention to the comorbid disorder, and clients tend to be extruded from both based on complications related to comorbidity. Treatment systems tend to be rigid at the interface and have difficulty developing and delivering care that is individualized and coordinated. Finally, in a parallel treatment model, there is often no fixed point of responsibility; the burden of integrating diverse aspects of the two systems typically falls to the client.

Many experts have recommended integrating treatment within one system for those with co-occurring severe mental disorder and substance use disorder (Carey, 1989; Drake, Bartels, Teague, Noordsy & Clark, 1993-a; Minkoff and Drake, 1991; Ridgely, Osher & Talbott, 1987; Teague, Schwab & Drake, 1990). A rational health care system would probably integrate mental health and substance abuse treatments at all levels (Little Rock Working Group, 1993), but the U.S. system did not develop for rational reasons and continues to be influenced by special interests that are relatively insensitive to the needs of dually diagnosed patients. Thus, for the immediate future, attempts to integrate treatment must be based on modifications of existing treatment systems.

In this chapter we will describe efforts to develop integrated treatments for the specific population of persons with co-occurring severe mental disorder and substance use disorder throughout one state mental health system since 1987. Other states have been engaged in similar efforts. What may make New Hampshire unusual in this regard is that a research team has been consistently involved in the effort to design, implement, and evaluate the system (Drake, Teague & Warren, 1990).

INTEGRATED TREATMENT

In integrated treatment, one group or team of clinicians addresses both disorders concurrently in the same setting (Drake et al., 1993-a). Integration implies much more than adding together two existing treatments; it produces a new synthesis of existing principles and techniques, and creates a hybrid group of clinicians who differ from current personnel in either system. For treating persons with severe mental disorders, integration within the existing mental health system rather than within the substance abuse treatment system is usually more efficient because the mental health system should already be providing the comprehensive treatment, support, and rehabilitative services that these individuals need (Bartels and Drake, 1991; Drake et al., 1993-a).

Research on Integrated Treatment

Limited research on integrating substance abuse treatments into mental health programs suggests that integrated treatment may be quite effective. Kofoed, Kania, Walsh and Atkinson (1986) and Hellerstein and Meehan (1987) found that dually diagnosed outpatients who participated in substance abuse treatment groups had lower rates of rehospitalization during one year of treatment. Ries and Ellingson (1990) found that attending inpatient drug and alcohol discussion groups was associated with abstinence for one month after discharge. Drake, McHugo and Noordsy (1993-b) found that over 60% of outpatients with co-occurring schizophrenia and alcoholism treated in an integrated outpatient program (described below) achieved stable abstinence within four years. Bond, McDonel, Miller and Penesec (1991) found that dually diagnosed clients treated in dual diagnosis groups in the mental health center reduced alcohol and marijuana use over 18 months.

In contrast to these positive results, Lehman, Herron and Schwartz (1993) found that a group of dually diagnosed clients treated with an integrated approach did not reduce their substance abuse over one year. According to the authors, the clients may not have been ready for active treatment and may have been followed too briefly.

A Statewide Dual-Diagnosis System

The New Hampshire system for persons with dual disorders was designed in 1987 by a joint effort of the New Hampshire Division of Mental Health, the state's Office of Alcohol and Drug Abuse Prevention, and the New Hampshire-Dartmouth Psychiatric Research Center (Drake et al., 1990; Drake, Antosca, Noordsy, Bartels & Osher, 1991-a). The system has been studied and refined since 1987 with support from the Robert Wood Johnson Foundation, the National Institute of Mental Health, and the National Institutes on Alcohol Abuse and Alcoholism. In the following sections, we will describe several components of the New Hampshire dual diagnosis system: assumptions, oversight, continuous treatment teams, dual diagnosis treatment groups, community mental health centers, inpatient care, residential care, family work, and training.

Assumptions: The system incorporates several key assumptions: that patients with severe mental disorders are the responsibility of the mental health system, that substance abuse treatment expertise should be integrated into the mental health system, and that a consistent focus on substance abuse should be provided at all levels of care — e.g., inpatient, outpatient, partial hospitalization, and residential. Another assumption is that treatment must match the explanatory models, level of awareness, and social skills of the individual client rather than that all clients must fit into one model of substance abuse and recovery. This follows from research on the heterogeneity of the population (see, e.g., Lehman, Myers & Corty, 1989) and the difficulty in using a traditional substance abuse treatment model with all clients (see, e.g., Drake et al., 1993-b).

The treatment system also recognizes that many of the patients are at a premotivational state, in which they are not acknowledging and seeking active treatment for their substance use disorders (Drake et al., 1990; Test, Wallisch, Allness & Ripp, 1989). Treatment must therefore proceed in a stage-wise fashion (Drake et al., 1991-a; Osher and Kofoed, 1989) as described in previous chapters: engagement stage, persuasion stage, active treatment and relapse prevention.

Oversight: At the beginning of the dual diagnosis initiative in New Hampshire, an advisory board was created that included clients, family members, clinicians, and representatives from the Department of Mental Health, the Office of Alcohol and Drug Abuse Prevention, and the Psychiatric Research Center. This board continues to meet regularly to review the development, maintenance, and evaluation of the statewide program. The Department of Mental Health (DMH) convenes the board, organizes the monthly training meetings (described below), contracts with mental health centers for dual diagnosis services, and monitors substance abuse at the client level through the mental health statistics improvement program. In addition, the Research Center staff meet weekly with the medical director of DMH to review the development and integrity of the program and to discuss using evaluation data for further refinements of the system. We have been fortunate that all of the major participants throughout the state have stayed in their positions, have maintained their commitment to the effort, and have cooperated in keeping the system flexible and protecting it from financial and other threats to validity.

Continuous treatment teams: In New Hampshire, the centerpiece of the integrated system is the continuous treatment team (CTT), a specialized team within each mental health center that takes primary responsibility for the care of a discrete caseload of dually diagnosed clients and secondarily for disseminating expertise on dual disorders throughout the center. Key features of the CTT model, which are used to evaluate model adherence, are as follows:

1. *Assertive engagement* CTTs assertively reach out to clients to develop a relationship, to help them engage in services, including mental health and substance abuse services, and to help them remain engaged. Assertive engagement includes visits to jails, hospitals, shelters, families, courts, and other settings where clients spend time. It also includes the ethical and appropriate use of legal mechanisms, such as payeeships, guardianships, conditional discharges, probation, and parole, to link clients with outpatient treatment and to prevent institutionalization. The goal of assertive engagement is to enable the client to manage his or her disorders and to make progress toward recovery over time.

2. *Provision of services in the community* CTTs meet with clients *in vivo* — i.e., in their living, working, and playing environments — as opposed to in the office or clinic. In these settings, they help clients to develop skills for daily living, socialization, structured activities, work, drug refusal, and family interactions. They also work directly with significant others, such as landlords, family members, roommates, and friends in the community to increase appropriate supports.

3. *Intensity* CTTs provide approximately two times the level of direct contact as traditional case management in New Hampshire. This level of intensity is maintained at least until the client has stabilized, usually until the client is in the relapse prevention stage, and can readily be reinstituted around relapses.

4. *Small caseloads* Caseloads are approximately ten clients per full-time clinician, excluding the psychiatrist's time. CTTs are expected to operate with a full complement of clinicians, with a caseload of the appropriate size, and without responsibilities to cover for other clinicians in the mental health center.

5. *Team approach* CTTs operate with a shared-caseload model rather than as a group of individual practitioners. Clients are assigned to an individual clinician only for the purpose of paperwork. CTT clinicians know all of the clients on the team, meet regularly with many clients, and devote more time to individual clients on the basis of the clients' needs and preferences. This allows clients to have access to a greater range of styles and expertise, and increases the likelihood of having a familiar person available during a crisis.

6. *Continuous responsibility* The CTT is responsible for a discrete group of clients 24 hours per day. The team provides direct coverage of all crises during daytime hours, and a team member is available by beeper at other times to ensure continuity of care and consistency of the treatment plan. The team arranges, coordinates, and participates in crisis care to ensure that hospitalizations are consistent with the plan. Because of intensive daytime services, most emergencies can be prevented.

7. *Collaboration with support system* CTT provides psychoeducational services to the client's family, significant others, friends, and supportive contacts, such as landlords and employers, as needed. This includes educating the family about substance abuse and linking them with mental health and substance abuse support groups. Support network members are regularly enlisted in carrying out behavioral plans. By providing attention and other rewards contingent upon appropriate behavior, they can avoid the frustration of reinforcing dysfunctional behaviors such as substance abuse and medication noncompliance. Family members and others are typically relieved and grateful for assistance that allows them to express their caring in a constructive fashion.

8. *Individualized substance abuse treatment* CTT provides individualized assessment and direct counseling for substance abuse problems.

All CTT clinicians become experts in substance abuse treatment, assess clients individually, and provide direct counseling that includes social network interventions, laboratory monitoring, and individual treatment plans. Interventions are individually designed to capitalize on clients' strengths and to use rehabilitation to promote positive lifestyle changes that will support and reinforce abstinence.

9. *Group treatment* CTT clinicians lead substance abuse treatment groups (described below) in the mental health center that are specifically designed for clients with dual disorders. Group treatment provides peer support, feedback, modeling, and validation for steps toward recovery from substance abuse. The group is a powerful intervention for those who can tolerate the group setting, and our work consistently shows that many clients who are unable to tolerate AA/NA groups are able to participate in dual diagnosis groups (Bartels and Thomas, 1991; Drake et al., 1993-b). These groups are described in more detail below.

10. *Dual diagnosis model* CTT uses a four-stage, dual diagnosis model of recovery, rather than the 12-step orientation. In the dual-diagnosis model, substance abuse treatment is highly individualized and non-confrontational; it follows behavioral principles, encourages understanding risk factors, helps clients to develop substitute behaviors and relationships, promotes medication compliance, and incorporates a rational understanding of the interactions between mental illness and substance abuse (Drake et al., 1993-a). Treatment avoids religious or abstract concepts and does not insist on immediate abstinence. The long-term goal in this model to promote a substance-free, satisfying lifestyle through social and vocational rehabilitation.

11. *Multidisciplinary team* CTTs include a half-time psychiatrist, a nurse, a substance abuse specialist, and at least one case manager, social worker, or other person experienced in the treatment or rehabilitation of persons with severe mental disorders. Critical components are integration of the psychiatrist and the nurse on the team and participation of at least one member with substance abuse treatment expertise. Generous team-meeting time promotes continuous supervision and cross-training.

12. *Continuity of staffing* CTTs ensure that clients have continuous relationships with the same staff over time. This necessitates not only a team approach but also minimal turnover of staff. The shared caseload model reduces turnover and the impact of any turnover that

does occur. Other factors that promote continuity of staffing include administrative support, the opportunity to try innovative approaches, development of dual diagnosis skills, and continuous training.

13. *Dual diagnosis specialization* CTTs are effective, confident, and enduring over time, in large part, because they become dual-diagnosis specialists with recognized expertise. In addition to working with their own clients and their families, team members can provide training, consultation, and liaison related to the treatment of dual disorders to other clinicians, other providers, and other stakeholders, such as family, police, and housing personnel. These functions are all consistent with their mission and expertise.

At the same time, CTT cannot solve all of the clinical problems in a mental health center, and diluting their mission or expertise by asking them to broaden their work too much may have disastrous consequences. Our experience indicates that the CTT caseload should include predominantly dual disorder clients rather than a mixture of clients who are difficult to treat for a variety of reasons. Experience has taught us that their expertise should include dual disorders defined as Axis I major mental illness plus substance use disorder. Other dually diagnosed groups, such as personality disordered patients who abuse substances and sex offenders who abuse substances, for example, may also need intensive services but need a substantially different approach that is not consistent with CTT.

Dual Diagnosis Groups

In all outpatient settings, CTT members lead weekly, peer-oriented, dual diagnosis groups. These include supportive, educational discussion groups that focus on the role of alcohol and drugs in patients' lives for those who are in the persuasion (or motivational) stage of treatment, and behaviorally-oriented, skill-training groups for patients who are in the active treatment stage (Noordsy and Fox, 1991). Persuasion and active treatment functions can be accomplished in the same group or in separate groups. Outreach and a variety of incentives are used to attract clients to regular attendance. The groups are open-ended, and clients often attend for one to two years. Some groups evolve into long-term support groups when the majority of members achieve the relapse prevention stage of treatment. Groups are typically led by two CTT clinicians, one with a mental health and one with a substance abuse treatment background.

Community Mental Health Centers

As described above, the CTT coordinates each center's dual diagnosis program, and their clinical expertise is transferred to the rest of the mental health center in several ways. First, the dual diagnosis group program, which is led by CTT, is offered to all appropriate clients in the center. This group can serve an assessment function for clients referred by other case managers. Second, CTT consults with other clinicians in the mental health center around training, evaluations, and treatment issues. When CTT functions well, we have found that their expertise spreads steadily throughout the center. Third, CTT provides liaison and training for staff in related programs, such as inpatient, partial hospitalization, housing, rehabilitation, and vocational. They also provide education and training to interested groups, such as lawyers, judges, police, probation and parole officers, and local educational programs.

Inpatient Care

Through outreach, consultation, and training, the dual diagnosis program has attempted to penetrate into all inpatient settings. The goal is to help inpatient units to increase their competence to assess and manage patients with co-occurring severe mental illness and substance use disorder. Since psychiatric inpatient admissions are usually brief and oriented toward acute stabilization, active education and treatment of substance abuse may not be appropriate for many clients. No consensus exists on this issue. Inpatient addiction treatment programs are typically too intensive and unable to adapt to the cognitive and social skill levels of most individuals with severe mental disorders. Poor retention and failure to transfer gains to the community are typical. Research evidence does not so far support using expensive inpatient resources for lengthy inpatient alcohol and drug treatment for this population (Drake et al., 1993-b). However, detection, assessment, treatment planning, and linkage with the outpatient dual-diagnosis system are always appropriate (see Drake and Mercer-McFadden in this volume).

Residential Care

Unstable housing is a consistent correlate of substance abuse in psychiatric patients (Drake, Wallach & Hoffman, 1989; Drake, Wallach, Teague, Freeman, Paskus & Clark, 1991-b), in part because housing programs and landlords require abstinence or extrude clients on the basis of substance abuse or associated disruptive behavior (see Dixon and Osher in this volume). This is equivalent to insisting on treatment success before offering treatment. A more realistic approach to housing might include providing professional supports as needed in all housing settings and perhaps a variety of housing situations, with different regulations regarding substance use, for dually diagnosed clients who are at varying stages of recovery and have different needs for structure, protection from the environment, and peer supports in their efforts to attain abstinence.

In the New Hampshire mental health system, we are working to develop and evaluate varying types of housing and supports. Since optimal housing arrangements for this population are as yet unclear, we encourage system managers to take an empirical, non-ideological approach to housing. For example, an initial attempt to provide residential treatment in a central setting for frequently rehospitalized clients was terminated because clients who attained sobriety there had such difficulty transferring their gains back to their community living settings (Bartels & Thomas, 1991). Of course, most clients are also supported in community apartments or family homes with attempts to guide them away from neighborhoods and cohabitants that promote substance abuse. Local alternatives for residential treatment, congregate living, and supported housing are currently being evaluated.

Working with Families

Even families that are well educated about severe mental disorders are often uninformed regarding alcohol and drug use disorders (Clark & Drake, 1992; Sciacca & Hatfield, in this volume). Families are included in the dual diagnosis program in a variety of ways. The mental health centers offer education, support, and skills training regarding substance abuse to families on a routine basis as part of a statewide psychoeducation program. CTT and other clinicians build on this program on an individualized basis. The CTTs in several centers also conduct multiple family groups that include families and clients. Finally, clients who have great difficulty controlling their substance use are sometimes helped by a behavioral plan that involves the family in providing their time and attention as positive reinforcers for sobriety in a contingent fashion.

Training

Training staff to work with dually diagnosed clients was our greatest challenge during the early years of developing the system. Since very few clinicians had any training in treating dual disorders in 1987, we needed to train our current workforce with a limited number of trainers (see Fox and Shumway chapter in this volume). The most successful experiences occurred in those mental health centers in which flexible, experienced clinicians from different backgrounds were allowed to struggle together to develop expertise and given the opportunity to present their difficulties to a variety of other clinicians both locally and at the CTT group meeting. Over time, the CTTs arrived together at a working model that is consistent within teams and across settings. The monthly meetings, which have occurred since 1988, include case discussions, talks by experts, and presentations of research data. In these meetings, teams learn from each other and develop agreements to visit each others' sites. For example, one CTT learned to extend the multiple family group method to dual diagnosis and began training the other CTTs when they had achieved some success. Similarly, one team that had greater initial success in starting their dual diagnosis group program provided training to the other teams. Now that the CTTs have achieved competence, we rely on monthly meetings to support each other in continuing to handle the most difficult clients. The teams themselves coordinate training in their local centers.

CONCLUSIONS

After six years of developing dual diagnosis expertise and programs on a statewide basis, clinicians, clients, and families are clearly more optimistic about the treatment of substance abuse in persons with severe mental disorders. As their skills have improved, clinicians have been more likely to detect substance abuse, to plan and implement an appropriate intervention within the mental health system, and to involve families and others effectively. Referrals to the traditional substance abuse system have decreased and almost disappeared. Clinicians and clients use the self-help system (AA/NA) with more realistic expectations. Families are also more likely to recognize substance abuse as a problem, to demand substance abuse education, and to expect more involvement in treatment. The clients are clearly recovering (Drake et al., 1993-b), and all of the major stakeholders continue to be involved in reviewing and improving the system.

REFERENCES

Bartels, S. J., & Drake, R. E. (1991). Dual diagnosis: New directions and challenges. *California Journal of the Alliance for the Mentally Ill. 2*, 6–7.

Bartels, S. J., & Thomas, W. N. (1991). Lessons from a pilot residential treatment program for people with dual diagnoses of severe mental illness and substance use disorder. *Psychosocial Rehabilitation Journal. 15*, 19–30.

Bond, G. R., McDonel, E. C, Miller, L. D., & Penesec, M. (1991). Assertive community treatment and reference groups: An evaluation of their effectiveness for young adults with serious mental illness and substance abuse problems. *Psychosocial Rehabilitation Journal. 15*, 31–43.

Carey, K. B. (1989). Emerging treatment guidelines for mentally ill chemical abusers. *Hospital and Community Psychiatry. 40*, 341–342.

Clark, R. E, & Drake, R. E. (1992). Substance abuse and mental illness: What families need to know. *Innovations and Research. 1*, 3–8.

Drake, R. E., Antosca, L., Noordsy, D. L., Bartels, S. J., & Osher, F. C. (1991-a). Specialized services for the dually diagnosed. In K. Minkoff & R. E. Drake (Eds.), *Dual Diagnosis of Major Mental Illness and Substance Disorder* (pp. 57–67). San Francisco: Jossey-Bass.

Drake, R. E., Bartels, S. J., Teague, G. B., Noordsy, D. L., & Clark, R. E. (1993-a). Treatment of substance abuse in severely mentally ill patients. *Journal of Nervous and Mental Disease. 181*, 606–611.

Drake, R. E., McHugo, G. J., Noordsy, D. L. (1993-b). Treatment of alcoholism among schizophrenic outpatients: 4-year outcomes. *American Journal of Psychiatry. 150*, 328–329.

Drake, R. E., Teague, G. B., & Warren, S. R. (1990). Dual diagnosis: The New Hampshire system. *Addiction and Recovery. 10*, 35–39.

Drake, R. E., Wallach, M. A., & Hoffman, S. (1989). Housing instability and homelessness among aftercare patients of an urban state hospital. *Hosptial and Community Psychiatry. 40*, 46–51.

Drake, R. E., Wallach, M. A., Teague, G. B., Freeman, D. H., Paskus, T. S., & Clark, T. A. (1991b). Housing instability and homelessness among rural schizophrenics. *American Journal of Psychiatry. 148*, 330–336.

Hellerstein, D. J., & Meehan, B. (1987). Outpatient group therapy for schizophrenic substance abusers. *American Journal of Psychiatry. 144*, 1337–1339.

Kofoed, L., Kania, J., Walsh, T., & Atkinson, R. M. (1986). Outpatient treatment of patients with substance abuse and coexisting psychiatric disorders. *American Journal of Psychiatry. 143*, 867–872.

Lehman, A. F., Herron, J. D., & Schwartz, R. P. (1993). Rehabilitation for young adults with severe mental illness and substance use disorders: A clinical trial. *Journal of Nervous and Mental Disease. 181*, 86–90.

Lehman, A. F., Myers, P., & Corty, E. (1989). Assessment and classification of patients with psychiatric and substance abuse syndromes. *Hospital and Commuity Psychiatry. 40*, 1019–1025.

Little Rock Working Group. (1993). Recommendations of the Little Rock Working Group on Mental and Substance Use Disorders in Health Care Reform. Little Rock, Arkansas: Center for Mental Healthcare Research.

Minkoff, K., Drake, R. E. (Eds.). (1991). *Dual diagnosis of major mental illness and substance disorder*. San Francisco: Jossey-Bass.

Noordsy, D. L., & Fox, L. (1991). Group intervention techniques for people with dual disorders. *Psychosocial Rehabilitation Journal. 15*, 67–78.

Osher, F. C., Kofoed, L. L. (1989). Treatment of patients with both psychiatric and psychoactive substance use disorders. *Hospital and Community Psychiatry, 40*, 1025–1030.

Regier, D. A., Farmer, M. E., Rae, D. S., Locke, B. Z., Keith, S. J., Judd, L. L., Goodwin, F. K. (1990). Comorbidity of mental disorders with alcohol and other drug abuse: results from the Epidemiologic Catchment Area (ECA) Study. *Journal of American Medical Association. 21*, 2511–2518.

Ridgely, M. S., Goldman, H. H., & Willenbring, M. (1990). Barriers to the care of persons with dual diagnoses: Organizational and financing issues. *Schizophrenia Bulletin, 16*, 123–132.

Ridgely, M. S., Osher, F. C., & Talbott, S. A. (1987). *Chronically Mentally Ill Young Adults with Substance Abuse Problems: Treatment and Training Issues*. Rockville, MD: Alcohol, Drug Abuse, and Mental Health Administration.

Ries, R. K., & Ellingson, T. (1989). A pilot assessment at one month of 17 dual diagnosis patients. *Hospital and Community Psychiatry 41*. 1230–1233.

Teague, G. B., Schwab, B., Drake, R. E. (1990). *Evaluating Services for Young Adults with Severe Mental Illness and Substance Use Disorders*. Arlington, VA: National Association of State Mental Health Program Directors.

Test, M. A., Wallisch, L. S., Allness, D. J., & Ripp, K. (1989). Substance use in young adults with schizophrenic disorders. *Schizophrenia Bulletin 15*. 465–476.

16

Human Resource Development

THOMAS S. FOX and DONALD SHUMWAY

The one segment of the field which must constantly adjust to changing trends and new realities is the mental health workforce. They are responsible for adapting to changing realities that affect where they work, what skills they will need on the job, how they can best provide the services, who they work with, and, even the philosophical under-pinnings that guide their efforts.

Fazzi, 1990

Since the early 1950's, the mental health field has experienced persistent and, at times, dramatic changes. The introduction of psychotropic drugs, the enactment of the Mental Health Centers Act of 1963, the deinstitutionalization movement of the 1970's, the advocates, family and consumer movements of the 1980's, and the ongoing development of viable community alternatives have all added to the changes. Many observers in the field think that the rate of change is even likely to increase. Changes in national health care policy, results of services research, renewed interest in research on antipsychotic medications, and other factors will only serve to accelerate changes. Therefore, to many who have worked in the mental health field for a number of years, it seems that the only durable reality is change. One area of significant change has been in the recognition that substance abuse is a common coexisting condition in severe mental illnesses (Ridgley, Goldman, & Willenbring, 1990; Minkoff & Drake, 1991) and that these coexisting conditions require a special workforce expertise in order to treat them.

This chapter is intended to assist practicing clinicians and program managers in developing a workforce to work with people with mental illnesses and substance use disorders amid all these fluctuating influences. The content of what they should know is contained in the other chapters of this book. This chapter will focus on the process of how to transfer emerging information into an existing workforce. This process must be seen as part of an overall commitment and strategy for training and retraining of professionals and paraprofessionals. Therefore, it is important to begin with an analysis of the essential components for any successful workforce development.

COMPONENTS OF SUCCESSFUL WORKFORCE DEVELOPMENT STRATEGY

Much has been written about personnel development and administration in mental health systems (Griffith, Cole, Small, & Phillips, 1992). In addition, extensive federal legislation over the last thirty years has either mandated or specified staffing and training requirements (Kent & Gibson, 1992). Perhaps the most useful and relevant information comes from the NIMH Mental Health Human Resource Development Program (Goodstein & Backer, 1991; Fazzi, 1990), which has over 20 years of experience in workforce development in a number of states with a variety of specialized projects (Carling, 1984). A number of useful concepts have emerged in this literature on Human Resource Development (HRD) that are applicable here. For this discussion, they are divided into the development and implementation phases.

Development Phase

Most important is a clearly identified and dedicated HRD staff at both a state and local level that can assess, facilitate, and evaluate the effectiveness of this new group of professionals. Because of the unique challenges presented with this particular workforce, a consistent and committed HRD staff is critical. Although change in programs and professional expertise can be realized quickly, program stabilization and updated information transfer will span years and requires this longterm commitment of specialized staff.

This HRD staff also must be able to advocate for a priority need without being compromised by responsibility for the system planning process itself. In many areas the HRD staff also have responsibility for the system plan as well. The importance of this HRD staff independence becomes more evident when working with this special population. Linkages with training institutions, public-academic organizations, other providers and trainers is imperative. Diluting this effort by having HRD staff also responsible for the overall planning process can result in the loss of precious time and resources (Goodstein & Backer, 1991).

Another critical developmental factor is HRD knowlegeability. HRD knowledgeability is a concept of education and awareness building in which state and local systems come to understand the importance of workforce development to overall organizational health. This can take the form of state or regional conferences, articles in employee publications, or consultations with various interested groups (state hospital directors, CMHC administrative staff, etc.). This concept is one of mutual support in which state, regional and local authorities buy into the need for an emphasis on the "human assets" of a system of care. This awareness becomes more evident when the need for the allocation or reallocation of resources arrives. Staff must be retrained and/or redeployed with predictable resistance, thereby requiring system awareness to support the change process.

Next, a set of goals must be articulated in writing. Timelines, resources, regional implementation, and people responsible should all be explicitly identified. These goals need to be integrated into a larger organizational plan wherever possible so as to eliminate gaps or duplication. In many ways, a systems approach is desirable. HRD is part of a larger framework of planning, development and services.

For example, working with people with mental illnesses and substance use disorders can result in a sense of urgency and frustration because of the high health and safety risks associated with dual conditions. The frustration comes when a workforce tries, based on this sense of urgency, and fails to intervene successfully. Without overall planning and coordination of a variety of services (eg. outpatient, inpatient, housing) along with the workforce changes, failure is likely. Therefore, the "system of care" must have the capacity to prioritize and support the development of its workforce and services accordingly.

Implementation Phase

The implementation phase of a specialized HRD process requires supportive circumstances. Access to technical assistance can be very useful. Although model programs are difficult to transfer (Bachrach, 1980; Bachrach, 1988), in the initial phases of implementation, working with others who operate a similar and successful program in a neighboring state supports the system change. Confidence in skills, optimism based on success, and realistic expectations begin to counter the negativism, frustration and resistance to change. The specifics of the change, however, must be resolved within the local, regional and statewide systems of care. Technical support can also demonstrate to administrative staff responsible for making funding and policy changes the workability of this kind of program change. Service demonstration projects, funded in a variety of ways, can also show effectiveness and success that can then stimulate change locally. In general, the closer a developing program is, geographically and programatically, to an existing successful program, the more likely the success. Transferring expertise from distant systems without adequate technical support will likely result in failure.

Openly acknowledging and anticipating a resistance to a workforce retraining and redeployment can actually reduce the resistance to change. People can talk about it directly and discuss real fears of job loss, lack of skills, and the consequences it may have for them personally. Mental health professionals are accustomed to hearing these concerns from their clients, but may experience some difficulty expressing their own anxieties, even in an open and supportive environment. Without this forum being held regularly, understandable behaviors and attitudes will arise that will, in effect, sabotage the change effort. Periodic meetings focusing on expected benefits and positive outcomes can significantly reduce resistance. Participation by management responsible for policy and funding in these forums will assure a much smoother transition.

No well planned workforce change can proceed without an appropriate commitment of resources. Underfunding the necessary training can result in staff frustration and burnout and, ultimately, program failure. Overfunding can result in the waste of precious resources. Therefore, accurately identifying resources, both financial and in-kind, is imperative. Based on the experience in states that have implemented successful programs for people with mental illnesses and substance use disorders (Drake, Antosca, Noordsy, Bartels & Osher, 1991; Ridgley, 1991; Fox, Fox & Drake, 1992), many mid-course corrections will be required. Therefore, flexibility in resource allocation/reallocation is needed. Another proven fiscal strategy consists of blending multiple funding flows. A combination of grants (research and service development), Medicaid, contracts for managed care, and state dollars is often needed until the new programs and staff become more solidified within the organization.

A frequent source of resources and support can come from a public-academic liaison (PAL). A PAL can provide a critical impact on workforce preparation, direction, and development. The PAL initiates students into the values and priorities of the public sector. A PAL brings together the professional personnel of academia with the service delivery systems of the public sector. This provides an excellent opportunity for applied service system research and evaluation. By carrying out research and evaluation with standardized data collection, uniform training and implementation, and outcome analysis, needed guidance is given to administrators and clinicians alike. If there is not an existing PAL, the development of this specialized workforce might present an opportunity and a focus to develop one. In any event, these kinds of programs have been useful, even critical, in providing the ongoing commitment necessary for change (Fox, Fox & Drake, 1992; Drake & Teague, 1990).

BARRIERS TO WORKFORCE DEVELOPMENT

Even with a viable workforce development and implementation plan, there are some barriers unique to this arena. Others have described these obstacles in detail (Ridgley et al., 1990; Talbott, Bachrach, & Ross, 1986).

In most models and systems of care currently described in the literature (Minkoff & Drake, 1991), the staff are retrained from an existing workforce. They usually come from either a mental health or a substance abuse background. Both of these fields have developed quite independently, have separate licensing and credentialing requirements, and often view each other skeptically. This has led to differences in treatment philosophy, terminology and organizational discontinuity. Programatically, Talbott et.al. (1986) noted that both structural and process deficits exist. This means that neither the appropriate range of services nor the continuity of care is likely. Simply knowing what to do and who will do it is insufficient. One must also know how to bridge these two workforce streams to develop a specialized or cross-trained group of providers (Drake, McLaughlin, Pepper & Minkoff, 1991).

In recent years, clinicians and researchers have advocated for a workforce that can treat the clients both concurrently and in an integrated way. Separate administrative structures for these personnel streams make this integration difficult. The seriousness of this divided responsibility should not be underestimated. This barrier is most easily illustrated from the consumers' point of view. They are often denied admission or discharged prematurely from the care they need and deserve. Organizations dealing with shrinking resources often institutionalize forms of service denial to limit unwanted exposure to underfunded programs. For example, the practice of determining the primary diagnosis of either substance abuse or mental illness means no continuity or integration of treatment for the client. This has been seen in other parts of the psychiatric system (Goldberg & Fogel, 1989). Mutual clients are viewed with the suspicion that they will drain precious resources needed to serve existing people.

With these various barriers in mind, and with a viable plan and process for workforce development, we can now turn to some specific suggestions for staffing and program needs for working with people with dual disorders.

DEVELOPING A CROSS-TRAINED WORKFORCE

Most observers advocate for a staff that can treat both the mental illness and the substance use disorder concurrently, with both conditions seen as deserving attention. This entails developing a cross-trained workforce that can integrate treatment philosophies, terminology, and language from both disciplines. At the same time, longterm plans must be put in place supporting the same level of integration in the pre-service education of staff. Curriculum reform, updated information based on current research, and input from the field will better prepare entry level staff graduating from institutions of higher education. However, the following suggestions focus more upon developing and refining a workforce in place.

First of all, there must be a single point of accountability for both staff development and client identification. The higher this accountability exists in a local, regional or state organization, the more likely the success of the programs. Wherever this single point exists, it must have the capacity and resources to identify clients appropriately and train staff accordingly. Linkages with other stakeholders must exist in order to resolve policy, eligibility, and funding problems as they arise.

Those expected to adopt this innovation must be convinced that the change will work. Furthermore, they must be aware of the program or practice. Information dissemination alone is usually not enough. Research on the dissemination and utilization of information spans decades and is summarized by Backer, (1991); Corrigan, McKain and Liberman,(1991); and Glaser, Abelson, and Garrison, (1983). Organizational and program decision makers must not only be held accountable, but must understand how the change will work. Expect these same people to also want to measure outcomes demonstrating the effectiveness and efficiency of the anticipated changes.

Both training streams, mental health and substance abuse, must be valued. Because of separate preparation, licensing and clinical training, professional suspicion and devaluation are predictable. The antidote to this potentially destructive process is to value both backgrounds and legitimize a process of learning from one another. Career ladders within the workforce should encourage additional training and credentialing from both disciplines. Implicit in this arrangement is the concept of developing treatment teams with representatives from both backgrounds.

Not only should the treatment teams represent mental health and substance abuse backgrounds, they should also be multi-disciplinary. The nature of this work is both complex and challenging. No single discipline currently possesses the skill range necessary to meet all of the clients' needs. Psychiatry, nursing, case management, vocational, substance abuse experts, and rehabilitation counselors all need to have input.

These teams, whether collaborative or integrated, should be allowed local flexibility and time to develop. With all of these disciplines and backgrounds, how they work together becomes critical. This process can be self-facilitated or directed externally. However, some team building process should be instigated before staff begin accepting caseloads. This process should be ongoing and mutually supportive as staff turn over or services expand.

Now is the time to begin the training/retraining of the identified staff. This can be accomplished in a number of ways including course work, seminars, study groups, technical consultations, and feedback from families and consumers. The initial input should be user-oriented, direct, and interactive in nature. Any combination of methods that accomplishes this kind of initial input is acceptable. This formal phase should be initiated prior to caseload assignments to facilitate group formation, professional trust, and the development of relevant clinical skills.

After the initial infusion of training and the beginning of assuming caseload responsibility, ongoing support and training must now be considered. This workforce quickly notices that they have lost their customary sources of professional support. They neither think nor talk like their peer group of origin. Although in an integrated team setting they can often derive some support from one another, this is often insufficient given the complexity and challenges of this work. Arrangements should be made to facilitate bringing teams or members of teams from adjacent regions together on a periodic basis. In these meetings staff may discuss problems in common, seek expert advice, or deal with the many controversies implicit in an emerging field of dual-diagnosis practice. But most importantly, they develop an extended peer group with which to identify and from which to derive support.

The other critical element in the need for ongoing training has to do with conflict resolution. Many of the practices in this emerging field of working with people with a dual diagnosis contradict traditional practice. If traditional practice would have been sufficient, the need to develop a new workforce would have been unnecessary. Therefore, professional conflict is both expected and facilitated. For example, someone with a mental health background may have been taught not to medicate anyone who is using substances abusively. Current research (Drake, Bartels, Teague, Noordsy & Clark, in press) however, emphasizes the importance of medicating a person's mental illness even while they are using substances abusively. On the other hand, someone with a substance abuse background may have difficulty working with a client who initially does not have abstinence from the abused substance as a goal. Again, current research supports engagement and persuasion over abstinence in the initial phases of treatment. These, and many other controversial issues will rapidly become the content of both the team process and the regional support groups. These settings also provide an opportunity for influential staff members to express enthusiasm for, and special recognition of the newly developing workforce.

No training and support would be complete without consumer and family input. The literature is filled with good ideas generated by professionals that failed when they met consumer or family feedback (Campbell, 1991; Maddy, Carpinello, Holohean & Veysey, 1991; Lebow, 1984; Tanzman & Yoe, 1989; Steinwachs, Kasper & Skinner, 1992). By building the likely recipients of the service into the ongoing training and support of the professionals, needless mistakes and irrelevancies can be avoided. Consulting with consumers and ex-consumers can also be helpful in assisting staff in the challenging phase of engagement into treatment. When possible, the team should think of having a trained ex-consumer as a member to assist in this ongoing task. Working with families and consumers can make the complex process of program and staff development run more efficiently and smoothly since the recipients of the service have been involved from the beginning.

Finally, the staff must be culturally and racially sensitive. Much has been written about implementing programs in an appropriate social and racial context (Green, 1982; Snowden, 1982; Wallen, 1992). Demographers predict that by the year 2060, "minorities" will outnumber Whites (Duke & Morin, 1991). In many urban settings, this is already the case. Therefore, it is important that the workforce reflect and are sensitive to the local cultural and racial mix. Some observers have shown how enhancing the cultural appropriateness of services to minorities can reduce the overall mental health care costs while improving the quality of care (Wallen, 1992).

CONCLUSION

A specialized workforce can be successfully developed to work with people with dual disorders and their families. This is done in the context of an established HRD strategy with a clear understanding of the barriers inherent in working with this clientele. Within this context a number of suggestions are offered based upon both experience and research. Following these suggestions assures the necessary administrative will to support the development of new clinical skills and programs to serve this often desperate and underserved population.

REFERENCES

Backer, T.E. (1991). *Drug abuse technology transfer*. Rockville, MD: National Institute of Drug Abuse.

Bachrach, L.L. (1980). Overview: Model programs for chronic mental patients. *American Journal of Psychiatry. 137*, 1023–1037.

Bachrach, L.L. (1988). On exporting and importing model programs. *Hospital & Community Psychiatry. 39*, 1257–1258.

Campbell, J.E. (1991). The consumer movement and implications for vocational rehabilitation services. *Journal of Vocational Rehabilitation. 1(3)*, 67–75.

Carling, P.J. (1984). Human resources for mental health: History, current status, and future directions of the National Institute of Mental Health's Center for State Human Resource Development. Burlington: University of Vermont.

Corrigan, P., McKain, S., & Liberman, R.P. (1991). Skills traing modules: A strategy for dissemination and utilization of rehabilitation intervention. In J Rothman, E Thomas (Eds.), *Intervention research*. Chicago: Haworth.

Drake, R.E., Antosca, L., Noordsy, D.L., Bartels, S.B., & Osher, F.C. (1991). New Hampshire's specialized services for people dually diagnosed with severe mental illness and substance use disorder. In K Minkoff, RE Drake (Eds), *Dual diagnosis of major mental illness and substance disorder*. (pp. 57–67). San Francisco: Jossey-Bass.

Drake, R.E., Bartels, S.J., Teague, G.B., Noordsy, D.L., & Clark, R.E. (1993), Treatment of substance abuse in severely mentally ill patients. *Journal of Nervous and Mental Disease. 181*, 606–611.

Drake, R.E., McLaughlin, P., Pepper, B., & Minkoff, K. (1991). Dual diagnosis of major mental illness and substance disorder: an overview. In K Minkoff, RE Drake (Eds), *Dual diagnosis of major mental ilness and substance disorder*. (pp. 3–12). San Fancisco: Jossey-Bass.

Drake, R.E., & Teague, G.B. (1990). State research structures: The New Hampshire-Dartmouth Psychiatric Research Center. *In Proceedings of the First Annual Conference of the National Association of State Mental Health Directors Research Institute*, (pp. 12–14). Arlington, VA, NASMHPD.

Duke, L., & Morin, R. (1991). Demographic shift reshaping politics. Washington Post, August 17, 1991.

Fazzi, R.A. (1990). Future perspectives in mental health. In *Human Resource Association of the Northeast*. Holyoke, MA.

Fox, T.S., Fox, M.B., & Drake, R.E. (1992). Developing a statewide service system for people with co-occuring mental illness and substance use disorders. *Journal of Innovations and Research. 1*(4), 9–15.

Glaser, E.M., Abelson, H., & Garrison, K.N. (1983). *Putting knowlege to use.* San Francisco: Jossey-Bass.

Goldberg, R.J., & Fogel, B.S. (1989). Integration of general hospital psychiatric services with freestanding psychiatric hospitals. *Hospital & Community Psychiatry. 40*:1057–1061.

Goodstein, J., & Backer T.E. (1991). *Strategic planning manual for mental health HRD system development projects.* Prepared for National Institute of Mental Health; Mental Health Human Resource Development Program.

Green, J.W. (1982). *Cultural awareness in the human services.* Englewood Cliffs, NJ: Prentice-Hall, Inc.

Griffin, E.E.H., Cole, R.A., Small, D.A., & Phillips, M.L., (1992). In Talbott, J.A., Hales, R.E., & Keill, S.L. (Eds), *Textbook of administrative psychiatry.* (pp. 253–286) Washington, DC: American Psychiatric Press, Inc.

Kent, J.J., & Gibson, R.W. (1992). In Talbott, J.A., Hales, R.E., & Keill, S.L. (Eds.). *Textbook of administrative psychiatry.* (pp. 239–250) Washington, DC: American Psychiatric Press, Inc.

Lebow, J. (1984). Comsumer satisfaction with mental health treatment. *Psychological Bulletin. 91*, 244–259.

Maddy, B.A., Carpinello, S.E., Holohean, E.J., & Veysey, B.M. (1991). Service and residential needs: Recipient and clinical perspectives. From New York State Office of Mental Health; Bureau of Evaluation and Services Research.

Minkoff, K., Drake, R.E. (Eds.) (1991). *Dual diagnosis of major mental illness and substance disorder*. San Francisco: Jossey-Bass.

Ridgley, M.S., (1991). Creating integrated programs for severly mentally ill persons with substance disorders. In K Minkoff, RE Drake (Eds). *Dual diagnosis of major mental illness and substance disorder*. (pp. 29–41). San Francisco: Jossey-Bass

Ridgley, M.S., Goldman, H.H., & Willenbring, M. (1990). Barriers to the care of persons with dual diagnoses: Organizational and financing issues. *Schizophrenia Bulletin. 16*:123–132.

Snowden, L. (Ed.) (1982). *Reaching the underserved: Mental Health Needs of Neglected Populations*. Beverley Hills, CA: Sage Publications.

Steinwachs, D.M., Kasper, J.D., & Skinner, E.A. (1992). Family perspectives on meeting the needs for care of severly mentally ill relatives: A national survey. Baltimore, MD: John Hopkins University School of Hygiene and Public Health, Center on the Organization and Financing of Care for the Severely Mentally Ill.

Talbott, J.A., Bachrach, L.L., & Ross, L. (1986). Non-compliance and mental health systems. *Psychiatric Annals. 16*, 596–599.

Tanzman, B., & Yoe, J. (1989). Vermont consumer housing and supports preference study. Burlington: University of Vermont, Center for Community Change Through Housing and Support.

Wallen, J. (1992). Providing culturally appropriate mental health services for minorities. *Journal of Mental Health Administration. 19*, 288–295.

17

Policy and Financing Issues in the Care of People with Chronic Mental Illness and Substance Use Disorders

M. SUSAN RIDGELY and LISA B. DIXON

Developing effective treatments for individuals with substance use disorders and mental illness requires expertise in overcoming complex obstacles in the domains of policy and financing. While convincing data about the effectiveness of innovative clinical programs can help to overcome these obstacles, workers at many levels of government and the private sector must also develop innovative strategies to modify the current care system. This chapter will describe barriers to effective treatment and then suggest models and strategies for change.

BARRIERS TO THE CARE OF DUALLY DIAGNOSED PEOPLE

There are a variety of impediments to developing systems of care to serve people with dual diagnoses. As has been discussed in previous chapters, these barriers include administrative discontinuities, resource constraints, distrust and philosophical conflicts among providers, and financing restrictions. Each of these serves to hinder or frustrate efforts to provide comprehensive care. Overcoming these barriers is key to the development of comprehensive systems of care for people with dual diagnoses.

Many States and localities lack a *common administrative structure* for alcohol, drug and mental health services. This is a hindrance to developing systems of care to serve people with dual diagnoses, for example, because there is no single *authority* to which all treatment systems are responsible. These service divisions are not an accident of history but reflect purposeful attempts to create structures to improve administrative efficiency. To ensure that categorical monies are spent for appropriate target populations, service systems set up eligibility requirements, usually focused on diagnosis. Particularly when funding is tight, utilization review and licensing standards are employed to ensure that only *eligible* individuals are served with categorical monies.

When people with multiple needs approach service systems, determining primary diagnosis is often one way of determining eligibility. This might result in one of two poor outcomes: identifying people as needing what an agency is able to provide (without reference to other needs) or identifying people as needing something another agency provides, as a way of denying access to services. Both are forms of institutional denial (Ridgely, Goldman & Willenbring, 1990).

People entering systems of care may also face another access problem. Those who request services are likely to be assigned to programs according to their presenting problems. Because mental disorders and substance use disorders are characterized by acute exacerbations, attention to immediate symptoms may not result in placement in the most appropriate program for the long term needs of the person.

Concerns about *scarce resources* have prevented extensive collaboration across service system boundaries. Requests for collaboration are often treated with concern that the result will be to take money from one system to pay for services for clients who are the responsibility of the other system.

Adding to this concern is a history of *distrust and philosophical conflicts*. These conflicts include disagreement, for example, about the use of psychotropic medication, the religious nature of Alcoholics Anonymous programs, and the appropriate role of recovering individuals as service providers in treatment programs (Minkoff, 1991).

Philosophical conflicts reflect the absence of a clinical consensus on appropriate treatment strategies across the service systems. To a certain extent, this may reflect different provider experiences. Many substance abuse service providers have treated people with primary substance use disorders who also suffer from anxiety or depression. They identify these people as dually diagnosed. By contrast, many mental health providers identify dually diagnosed population as people with severe mental disorders and substance abuse problems. It is not difficult to understand why there is no clinical consensus about how to treat persons with "dual diagnosis." In addition, there are a multiplicity of views within each field about the nature of these disorders and philosophies of intervention. To some extent these views represent the differential training and credentialing of the two fields. These philosophical conflicts, fueled by a lack of information about the other field and lack of respect for one another's competencies, have exacerbated the barriers between the systems of care.

Finally, and perhaps most pervasively, there are *financial barriers* to the care of dually diagnosed persons. In most States, providers are licensed and receive public monies exclusively to provide either mental health or substance abuse treatment services. In most cases public funding, provided through grant or contract mechanisms, is allocated to the agency to provide specific units of service to eligible clients. Agencies typically have no authority to co-mingle funds from a variety of funding streams and there are few agencies that meet the administrative requirements (e.g., licensing, building codes, staffing standards) to provide both mental health and substance abuse treatment services. In many cases these rules and requirements are conflicting so that attempting to provide integrated services would cause a single agency to come under the regulatory control of more than one State or local administrative authority.

Issues of third party payment are even more complex. For some individuals, having a history of mental illness or substance abuse may prevent them from being eligible for coverage by third-party payers. If individuals are qualified for coverage, they must then gain access to services. Often the services designed to treat dually diagnosed individuals are not covered by insurance or are only covered with strict limits.

Many assume that those who do not have access to private insurance will be treated in the public sector. It is also assumed that they will qualify for disability benefits, making them eligible for public health care benefits as well. For example, they may qualify for disability benefits from the Veteran's Administration (VA) or the Social Security Administration (SSA). The disabled veteran gains access to the VA health care system via VA disability, and the SSA disabled individual generally gains access to Medicare or Medicaid. Qualifying for these programs, however, is more complicated and less certain for the individual who suffers from dual diagnoses. Access to disability programs may be severely limited for people disabled by substance use disorders. Both the VA and SSA have special restrictions on benefits. Recipients may be denied benefits for failing to continue in treatment, even though the only available treatment is inappropriate to their needs. Claimants with dual diagnoses may need to qualify for benefits under the criteria for schizophrenia or some other non-substance use related disorder.

Apart from its impact on access to care, the proliferation of multiple providers funded by multiple sources, including public and private insurance, has resulted in a patchwork rather than a system of care. Each agency is free to decide which individuals to accept into services and what services to provide, and these decisions are often based more on the availability of financing than on client needs and preferences. Most agencies will provide those services for which the local mental health and substance abuse authorities are willing to pay, but they will provide those services according to their own policies and procedures, resulting in certain clients being excluded even from publicly funded services.

Given these barriers, the consumer seeking assistance and treatment may experience frustration, anger, and perhaps hopelessness. In addition to coping with their mental and substance use disorders, they must struggle to obtain treatment, housing, health care, and employment, a situation that may exacerbate their illnesses and further diminish their quality of life.

ORGANIZING A SYSTEM OF CARE

In many communities the system of care to provide services for people with mental or substance use disorders resembles less a system than a geographic cluster of agencies. Often there is no local authority fostering a "big picture" understanding of agencies as part of a larger system, with varying roles and responsibilities in that system. In most communities, there are alcohol and other drug treatment agencies, mental health agencies, and other human service agencies that provide services to dually diagnosed people. The agencies within each of these fields may or may not have collaborative relationships with other agencies within their own fields. For instance, many commentators have written about the lack of coordination and collaboration within the mental health field (Mechanic & Aiken, 1987). The descriptor *system* implies that there is some interrelationship among these agencies and across the fields. In many communities there is little if any active involvement across these boundaries.

One way to distinguish a community that has a *system of care* is that such a community offers a *continuum of services* and those services working together provide for *continuity of care* for people with severe mental illnesses. As Talbott, Bachrach and Ross (1986) have observed, local service systems can fail their clients and ultimately their communities in one of two ways. First, a local community system may have *structural deficits* — they may lack an appropriate range of alternative services for people with mental health and substance abuse problems. Second, the community system may suffer from *process failures*. Even though all the relevant services are available, the system does not provide continuity of care. Often it is easier to develop consensus on the development or modification of treatment interventions (addressing structural deficits) than it is to develop consensus on system changes that will address process failures.

Before addressing either the structural or process issues, a key decision to be made in organizing a system of care for people with dual diagnoses concerns the system's locus of control — will it be under the auspices of the local mental health authority, the local substance abuse authority, or a local human services authority? Though treatment ideologies often determine which system assumes leadership, ideology may be less important than funding, licensing and operating issues discussed above. Specialized programs have developed both within mental health and substance abuse authorities, though it is more common for mental health authorities to take responsibility when the population of interest has been severely mentally ill people with substance abuse problems (Ridgely,

Osher & Talbott, 1987). Whichever authority takes control, the system must be able to access the full range of services across the spectrum of service systems.

Addressing the structural issues first, many commentators have written about the need for a continuum of community-based services for treatment and rehabilitation of severely mentally ill people. The idea of a continuum of services is not meant to imply that every client receives every service in some sort of prearranged sequence, but rather that clients may be expected to need access to a range of supports to meet their individualized treatment and rehabilitation needs.

There are a number of ways that people working together in a community can develop such an array of appropriate programs to serve dually diagnosed people. *Existing programs* providing mental health and substance abuse treatment services can be adapted or modified to provide for the special needs of people with dual diagnoses. In order for adaptation to make sense as a strategy, there must be an ample number of quality mental health and substance abuse programs available in the local community. In the alternative, depending on the quality and adequacy of existing programs, *new integrated programs* specially targeted to people with dual diagnoses can be developed (see Chapter 15). In making the decision whether to adapt existing programs or develop new programs a number of factors may be considered, chief among those are the *flexibility* of local programs (and program providers) and financial resources.

STRUCTURE: THREE APPROACHES

There are three models for addressing the structural aspects of services integration for people with dual diagnoses: (1) the integrated service model; (2) the parallel service model; and (3) the linkages service model. Each has distinct strengths and weaknesses.

The Integrated Service Model

The integrated service model provides for the treatment of both mental health and substance use problems within a single service setting. The potential benefit of this approach is the opportunity for clinicians trained in both mental health and addictions to provide simultaneous treatment for both disorders in a setting specifically designed for this purpose (Minkoff, 1991). The major weakness of the integrated service model is a pragmatic one:

> a significant problem with this model [however] is the difficulty of developing sufficient numbers and varieties of hybrid programs to accommodate both the numbers of dual diagnosis patients and the variations in their diagnoses, levels of acuity, levels of disability, and degree of motivation (Minkoff, 1991).

The Parallel Service Model

The parallel service model, by contrast, allows for the use of existing treatment programs in both the alcohol and drug and mental health fields. While this approach may be more acceptable pragmatically, it puts the burden of coordinating care on the clients rather than on the agencies. In developing a system of parallel treatment, most of the focus is on accessibility.

This approach assumes that there are adequate substance abuse and mental health programs in the community. The problem is defined as one of identifying the needs and preferences of clients and matching them with an existing program or programs that can meet those needs and preferences. People with dual diagnoses would be referred to both mental health and substance abuse programs to receive treatment concurrently or sequentially.

Proponents of parallel treatment counsel that this approach allows clients to access more "normalizing" addiction treatment experiences, such as AA groups (Minkoff, 1991). The major drawback of this approach is the burden it places on the client or case manager "to maintain continuity though multiple episodes of treatment in diverse programs in distinct systems of care" (Minkoff, 1991; see also Drake, Osher & Wallach, 1991; Ridgely et al., 1987; (NIMH, 1992).

The Linkages Service Model

The linkages service model has been proposed by Kline and his colleagues specifically for homeless people with co-occurring disorders

(Kline, Harris, Bebout & Drake, 1991). This model is a composite of the integrated and parallel models and applies equally well to domiciled dually diagnosed persons. The linkages model provides for all mental health treatment to be offered within one integrated program but the substance abuse treatment to be provided by outside substance abuse agencies.

Clinical case managers are the key to the linkages with substance abuse agencies. Case managers identify, refer, and aggressively monitor services provided by the substance abuse agencies, as well as support their clients' use of AA and other self-help organizations. Case managers are expected to maintain collaborative relationships with substance abuse providers, educating them about severe mental illnesses and psychotropic medications (Kline et al., 1991).

Kline and his colleagues propose three strengths of this model for serving homeless dually diagnosed people: (1) Many homeless people have already made AA connections through shelters and other programs. This model enhances those linkages rather than imposing new therapeutic relationships. (2) The intensive case management approach emphasizes community outreach and is less stigmatizing and more acceptable than traditional services. (3) The emotional intensity of integrated programs may overwhelm home- less people, causing "flight" from the programs. As with parallel treatment, the major weakness is that this model cannot insure that appropriate substance abuse treatment, responsive to the clinical needs and preferences of the client, is actually delivered (Kline et al., 1991).

These models are not mutually exclusive. It is possible that within one comprehensive service system there are some integrated treat- ment programs, as well as a variety of other programs modified to be more appropriate for, and accessible to, homeless people with dual diagnoses.

PROCESS: ASSURING CONTINUITY OF CARE

Beyond the structural elements of a continuum of care are so-called process issues — those aspects of the system that provide for con- tinuity of care. Continuity of care has been defined as "a process in- volving the orderly, uninterrupted movement of patients among the diverse elements of the service delivery system" (Bachrach, 1981).

Simply having access to a variety of mental health or substance abuse programs will not insure that clients receive the care they need.

In organizing a system of care, it is necessary to consider how the various clinical components will fit together into a systemic approach to treatment and rehabilitation. According to Bachrach (1981), there are seven important dimensions of continuity of care. For care to be described as continuous, it must be *longitudinal* — the treatment must continue even though specific sites and caregivers may change over time. Care must also be *individualized*, planned with the client, and if the client desires, with their family, as well. Continuous care is also *comprehensive* and *flexible*, responding to changes in the client's needs and preferences over time. Relationships are important to continuous care, making such care *personal*. Finally, continuous care is *accessible* and *cohesive*. Barriers are removed or reduced, and there is a link among all service providers within the system of care. Case management may play a big role in assuring that clients receive the care they need and desire.

In beginning to think of a system of care, rather than specific clinical programs, it is important to consider how clients will enter the system and who will match them to an appropriate program according to their needs and preferences. In most communities, clients may enter a system through a number of public or private agencies in both the mental health and substance abuse treatment sectors or may become known to the system through emergency rooms or jails. Assignment is often done after preliminary assessment by the program or institution with which the client first comes into contact. Because providers tend to view individuals as having *either* mental illness or a substance use disorder, many people are denied care when they do not fit the eligibility criteria of a particular agency, or they are accepted by an agency when their needs may be better served by another program. Both of these situations are less than optimal.

If the entry and assessment functions were centralized, people who are suspected of having a dual diagnosis could be better matched to appropriate treatment programs. Centralization may mean that one agency provides all assessment and helps clients choose a program or programs for care, or it may mean that each agency reports its assessment to a central authority if it accepts a client into care. If the client is not to be served in that agency, the provider can make either a general or specific referral to another agency through a central "clearinghouse."

There is no definitive assessment strategy useful in classifying people with co-occurring disorders and assigning them to appropriate treatment options (Lehman, Myers & Corty, 1989). In addition, many smaller agencies are unable to provide comprehensive assessment and evaluation for people in acute psychiatric or substance-induced crises. Since it is the crisis phase that often leads to an individual being assigned to treatment, it is important that a system be able to handle crises, make initial assessments, match clients to caregivers, and adjust treatment plans over time to respond to each client's ongoing and changing needs. Because initial, comprehensive assessment is often an expensive undertaking, centralization would make it more affordable.

In viewing the care of dually diagnosed people from a process perspective, it is important for a system to decide who will provide what services and how they will be financed. For instance, if the community believes that detoxification is an important service, should it be provided in a hospital or is non-medical (or social) detoxification acceptable? Which agencies in the community are the best equipped to handle this service? If Medicaid funding is not available for detoxification services, how will the services be financed? Because there is often a gap between 24-hour care and aftercare in which many clients are lost to the system, how will that gap be handled? Is discharge planning and implementation the responsibility of the hospital staff?

As mentioned previously, many agencies depend on case managers to provide continuity of care by providing the linkage between the clients and the agency or agencies from whom they receive services. However, definitions of case management vary widely (Willenbring, Ridgely, Stinchfield & Rose, 1991) and most often case managers work for specific agencies, meaning that their reach only goes as far as the agency's connection with the client. If case managers are to represent the interests of the client and provide a focal point for continuity of care in the system, there is an argument to be made that case managers should operate system-wide, rather than being employees of each agency.

Rather than attempting a more comprehensive structural solution, many systems of care have focused on case management as the solution to problems of continuity of care (Willenbring et al., 1991), depending on case managers both to provide assertive outreach to engage people into services and to provide the linkage between the clients and the agency or agencies from whom they receive services. As Mechanic (1989) has warned, however:

> Case-management is loosely thought of as a solution to a wide variety of difficult problems. But the responsibilities it is expected to bear are alarming in the context of the realities of system disorganization and the types of personnel given these tasks.... Thus, case-management, to be effective, must be embedded in an organizational plan that defines clearly who is responsible and accountable for the care of the most highly disabled patients, has in place the necessary service elements to provide the full spectrum of needed services, and can coordinate and control diverse resources that flow into the system so that balanced decisions can be made about the expenditure of limited resources.

When there are no structural deficits and no process failures, a community could be described as having an effective system of care. More importantly, a service system may be described as being effective when people with dual diagnoses can access an appropriate array of services and opportunities that they feel meet their needs.

STRATEGIES FOR SYSTEMS INTEGRATION

Comprehensive systems of care for special needs populations are largely developed at the local level. However, because State governments influence local communities, often either enhancing or restricting their ability to be innovative, changes at the State level may strengthen or reinforce local efforts at services integration.

State Initiatives

There are a number of ways in which States can help local communities improve systems of care for people with co-occurring disorders. State agencies can help local communities by making people with dual diagnoses a priority in their State plans, funding new services, sponsoring training and evaluation, and promoting activities designed to enhance local system flexibility. In particular, leadership at the State level may be a necessary step to demonstrate and encourage collaboration among mental health, alcohol, and drug abuse agencies at the local level.

Some States have engaged in joint program development across State agencies and/or have published Requests for Proposal for jointly funded programming to serve people with co-occurring disorders. Others have established (and modeled) working agreements between and among State agencies. These agreements have been established for data collection, planning, and program development (Ridgely, et al., 1990). State agencies working together across the barriers of service systems can enhance local program development by, for example, developing guidelines for local authorities and providers to use in establishing appropriate services for people with dual diagnoses.

One of the most significant effects that State agencies could have on the development of improved systems of care in local communities would be to erase some of the categorical funding barriers that make it difficult to finance innovative programs. For example, the State mental health and substance abuse authorities could work with the State Medicaid agency to modify Medicaid programs to fund a range of community-based options for people with dual disorders. Both benefit limits and payment limits are at issue. Unless reimbursement rates for services to people with co-occurring disorders are modified, the tendency under current cost containment constraints will be for people with special needs to be underserved (Ridgely et al., 1990).

In addition, State agencies must recognize that there are increased costs associated with the care of people with dual diagnoses, and that the reimbursement rates for such specialized programs need to provide incentives to deliver quality services. The situation in many States today is the opposite. Many providers are struggling to manage the increased costs of treating two disorders within the reimbursement from one State agency. For example, many mental health programs are attempting to add substance abuse treatment components to their services without any additional funding from either the State mental health or substance abuse agency.

Regulatory barriers can also inhibit program development. State agencies can help, for example, by waiving exclusion criteria, licensure requirements, and staffing requirements to allow new programs to be developed. Separate, more flexible criteria for programs serving people with dual diagnoses may need to be created. States also can help support innovation by providing local authorities with training opportunities and technical assistance in developing and enhancing programs for underserved populations.

Local Initiatives

There are a number of ways in which a local community can create a system of care to serve people with dual diagnoses. These strategies range from actual change in the governance of systems of care to strategies for improved coordination of financing and delivery of care without structural change. The pros and cons of each strategy, as well as its applicability to local conditions, should be considered. Perhaps the most ambitious proposal is the development of one local authority with clear responsibility for serving the target population.

Local mental health authority: A local mental health authority centralizes all administrative, fiscal, and clinical control for services to people with severe mental illnesses in a city or county area (see Table 17.1). One example is the development of local mental health authorities required by the Robert Wood Johnson (RWJ) Foundation Program on Chronic Mental Illness (Shore & Cohen, 1990; Goldman, Morrissey & Ridgely, 1990). In describing the Foundation's rationale for creating such authorities, Shore and Cohen (1990) write:

> These successful programs [programs with a centralized mental health authority] share several elements: a comprehensive range of services and programs ensuring appropriate care for people at various stages of illness and disability ... assignment of clearly defined and continuing responsibility for each client with chronic mental illness, whether in the hospital or community; and budgetary control over all relevant services and settings, with fiscal incentives for providing appropriate and cost-effective care.

Each of the nine cities in the Foundation's demonstration implemented the concept of a centralized mental health authority differently, but in each case changes in philosophy, planning, and governance of the system of care were achieved, though generally the changes exceeded the financial capacity of the system to produce the desired levels of clinical change.

Table 17.1. Local Public Mental Health Authorities

Elements

---

1. Recentralization of the fiscal, administrative, and clinical control to a local county, city, or independent authority.

2. Responsibility for all persons eligible for public programs in a defined geographic area.

3. Responsibility for the full range of services required by this population, including general hospital inpatient care, state mental hospital system care, outpatient services, rehabilitation services, special residential housing needs, day treatment, and other related programs.

4. Fiscal responsibility for the cost of state mental health care by its eligible population (no pass-through of these costs to the state mental health budget).

5. Pooling of all funds (state mental health authority, Medicaid, and so on) to create a prospective annual budget.

6. Authority to retain savings and reprogram such savings at the discretion of the system.

7. Fiscal risk for overruns, although leniency is usually observed by the state mental health authority.

8. Authority to disperse funds by contract, grant, or direct provision of care, in whatever mix is optimal for local circumstances.

Source: Taube, Goldman & Salkever (1990).

The most important strength of this approach is the clear focus of authority and responsibility within one organizational structure. Each mental health authority controls the entire system of care, including the funding of all services. The potential downside of this strategy is the time and enormous amount of energy that must be devoted to reorganization at the highest levels of local government. The preliminary evaluation of the RWJ program found that it took each site a minimum of two years to put a local mental health authority in place (Goldman et al., 1990). In addition, serving people with dual diagnoses may require the consolidation of alcohol, drug, and mental health services into one local authority to assure appropriate care. While this would be a more difficult undertaking, it is not impossible at the local level. One of the RWJ demonstration authorities (Columbus, Ohio) has control of alcohol, drug, and mental health services throughout Franklin County (Goldman, Morrissey, Ridgely, Frank, Newman & Kennedy, 1992).

Both within and outside of the RWJ demonstration, there are a variety of models for organizing services, some through government agencies, non-profit organizations, and boards. None has exemplified clear strengths over the others and, in fact, local conditions (such as the existence and strength of local providers and the local political climate) factor heavily in the determination of how service systems might be organized (Goldman et al., 1992).

Other strategies: It may be neither necessary nor prudent to attempt to change the governance of the various systems of care needed to provide comprehensive services to people with dual disorders. There are a number of other mechanisms that have been used at the local level to improve systems of care. These include promoting joint planning (exemplified in service clusters), improving referral networks, creating interagency agreements and providing opportunities for cross training.

Service clusters: Where centralization of authority within a single local authority is not feasible, such as in children's services where so many different public and private agencies are participating, a form of joint planning and service provision called a *service cluster* has been used. A service cluster is composed of the public organizations that fund care for a specific population and the public and private agencies that provide care for a specific target group. The funders agree to share the cost of care determined to be necessary, and the agencies providing services agree to a common treatment plan and to sharing information.

Service clusters, and joint planning in general, only work if all relevant agencies agree to participate in the process. It is important that all local authorities and agencies, as well as consumers and family members, be included early in the planning process. In the case of people with dual diagnoses, this would include local mental health, substance abuse, human service and housing providers. If the plans do not represent a consensus of all agencies concerned, the effort may ultimately fail.

Referral networks: A second strategy is to improve referral networks, especially those across the boundaries of the alcohol, drug abuse, and mental health systems. It is common knowledge that clients "fall through the cracks" when they are referred from one agency to another. Referral networks can be improved by instituting some standard procedures (a common form, an agreement about sharing information) and by providing assistance in the referral process. In addition, many local communities use case managers to bridge the gaps between agencies. For case managers to be able to bridge gaps across service systems, however, their authority must be recognized by all the service systems. Case managers should not be put in the position of being "professional beggars," attempting to place people in agencies that have no obligation or interest in serving them. As Mechanic (1989) has noted, "case managers typically do not have the training and experience, control over resources, or professional standing to command resources from other organizations or even be persuasive with them." On the other hand, the directors of these agencies do have the power and authority. Interagency agreements may be necessary to enhance the process.

Interagency agreements: Such efforts may be more effective if they begin at the top, with interagency agreements between authorities or agencies. These agreements can be used to set policy (e.g., outlining an open door policy among agencies serving dually diagnosed people), to alter staffing patterns (e.g., detailing substance abuse staff to work part-time in a mental health agency), and to change clinical practice (e.g., setting out procedures for cross-agency collaboration on the clinical care of individual clients).

One of the goals of these mechanisms is to develop and then to institutionalize new ways of delivering care to people with dual diagnoses. Because it is easier to innovate than to maintain a new way of doing business, program administrators and staff will need to keep lines of communication open. This will help prevent misunderstandings that may result from traditional philosophical differences between the alcohol, drug, and mental health fields and insure that new ways of doing business are not eroded through neglect. It is important that agencies adopt a method of conflict resolution so that problems can be resolved quickly.

Cross-training: Finally, cross-training of staff is critical to the success of attempts to integrate care for people with dual diagnoses. One of the reasons that cross-training has gained popularity is that it makes use of currently available expertise and provides an opportunity for staff of mental health, alcohol, and drug treatment agencies to meet and work together in a non-threatening environment. Such programs should impart information and also be designed to build skills and competency. If handled correctly, joint meetings may provide an opportunity to air some of the differences in treatment philosophy that often separate the fields of alcohol, drug, and mental health treatment.

State authorities may need to help fund additional training for all staff that focuses on the special needs of people with dual diagnoses, preparing clinicians to address the practical issues faced by caregivers in either system. Two other groups can be very helpful in training staff. Homeless service providers can participate in addressing the difficulties of working with people on the streets and in shelters. Consumers can provide perspective on all aspects of service delivery and indicate how services could be made more "user friendly."

CONCLUSION

What are the critical elements of an integrated system for people with dual diagnoses? Several commentators have emphasized the need for attention to the clinical aspects of care as well as the integration of systems of care (Drake et al., 1991; NIMH, 1992; Minkoff, 1991). To paraphrase from these commentaries, to be an effective system of care there must be increased clinical capacity of individual clinicians to treat both severe mental illness and substance use disorders. In addition, there must be a range and variety of quality clinical programs to provide care to a heterogeneous population with diverse clinical needs. These programs must be integrated in some way into one overall system of care. While some commentators express a preference for reorganization of the structure of government in local communities, others advocate that integration can be accomplished by such mechanisms as service clusters and service coalitions, as long as there is a shared view of the respective roles and responsibilities of each partner in the system, and as long as there is a lead authority for the system at the local community level. It is generally agreed that there must be some coordination of administration, monitoring and funding at the State level to enhance, rather than stifle, innovation. Finally, the Federal and State governments can enhance resources and provide technical assistance to help local communities figure out what must be done and how to do it.

It must be said, in conclusion, that it is no mystery that most communities turn to case management rather than structural change to solve the problems of dysfunctional systems. This approach preserves the status quo and ultimately puts the burden of integration on clients, and their case managers, rather than on the system of care. However, it is not realistic for local communities to expect case managers to accomplish at the client level what they refuse to tackle at the system level. Solving the problem of fragmented care will take all the creativity and flexibility that communities can muster. The rewards, however, are well worth the struggle.

REFERENCES

Bachrach, L. (1981). Continuity of care for chronic mental patients: A conceptual analysis. *American Journal of Psychiatry. 138*, 1449–1455.

Drake, R., Osher, F., & Wallach, M. (1991). Homelessness and dual diagnosis. *American Psychologist. 46*, 1149–1158.

Goldman, H., Morrissey, J., & Ridgely, M.S. (1990). Form and function of mental health authorities at RWJ Foundation program sites: Preliminary observations. *Hospital and Community Psychiatry. 41*, 1222–1230.

Goldman, H., Morrissey, J., Ridgely, M.S., Frank, R., Newman, S., & Kennedy, C. (1992). Lessons from the Program on Chronic Mental Illness. *Health Affairs. 11*, 51–68.

Kline, J., Harris, M., Bebout, R., & Drake, R. (1991). Contrasting integrated and linkage models of treatment for homeless, dually diagnosed adults. *Dual Diagnosis of Major Mental Illness and Substance Disorder*. New Directions for Mental Health Services, No. 50, San Francisco: Jossey-Bass.

Lehman, A., Myers, P., & Corty, E. (1989). Assessment and classification of patients with psychiatric and substance abuse syndromes. *Hospital and Community Psychiatry. 40*, 1019–1024.

Mechanic, D. (1989). Central perspectives in formulating mental health policies. *Mental Health and Social Policy*, Third Edition. Englewood Cliffs, NJ: Prentice Hall.

Mechanic, D., & Aiken, L. (1987). Improving the care of patients with chronic mental illness. *New England Journal of Medicine. 317*, 1634–1638.

Minkoff, K. (1991). Program components of a comprehensive integrated care system for seriously mentally ill patients with substance disorders. *Dual*

Diagnosis of Major Mental Illness and Substance Disorder. New Directions for Mental Health Services, No. 50, San Francisco: Jossey-Bass.

National Institute of Mental Health. (1992). Outcasts on Main Street: Report of the Federal Task Force on Homelessness and Severe Mental Illness. Rockville, MD: National Institute of Mental Health.

Ridgely, M.S., Goldman, H., & Willenbring, M. (1990). Barriers to the care of persons with dual diagnoses: Organizational and financing issues. *Schizophrenia Bulletin. 16*, 123–132.

Ridgely, M.S., Osher, F., & Talbott, J. (1987). *Chronic mentally ill young adults with substance abuse problems: Treatment and training issues*. Baltimore: University of Maryland at Baltimore, School of Medicine, Mental Health Policy Studies.

Shore, M., & Cohen, M. (1990). The Robert Wood Johnson Foundation Program on Chronic Mental Illness: An overview. *Hospital and Community Psychiatry. 41*, 1212–1216.

Talbott, J., Bachrach, L., & Ross, L. (1986). Non-compliance and mental health systems. *Psychiatric Annals. 16*, 596–599.

Taube, C., Goldman, H., & Salkever, D. (1990). Medicaid and mental illness. *Health Affairs, 9*, 5–18.

Willenbring, M.L., Ridgely, M.S., Stinchfield, R., & Rose, M. (1991). *Application of case management in alcohol and drug dependence: Matching techniques and populations*. (DHHS Pub. No. ADM 91-1766). Rockville, MD: National Institute on Alcohol Abuse and Alcoholism.

Index